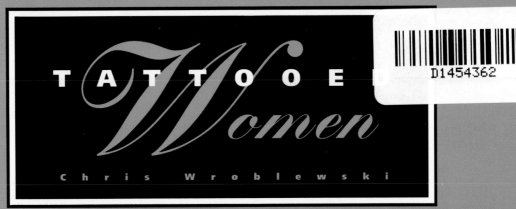

TATTOOED Women

Chris Wroblewski

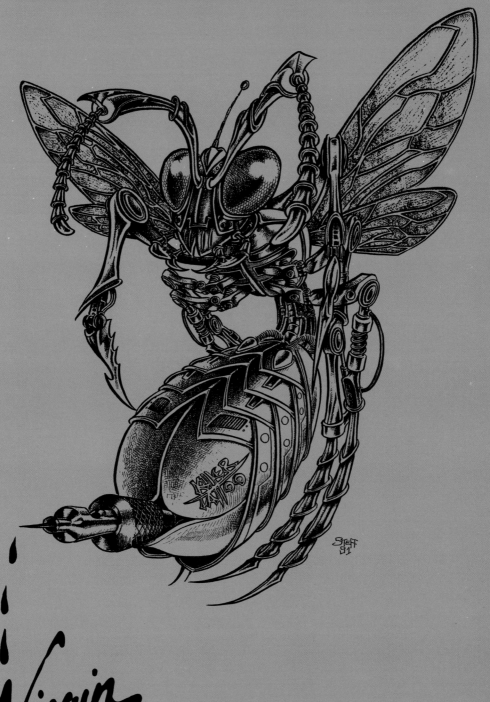

STEFF
91

Virgin

A Virgin Book
Published in 1992 by Virgin Publishing Ltd
338 Ladbroke Grove
London W10 5AH

A catalogue record of this book is available from the
British Library

Designed by Planet 'X'

Printed in Singapore

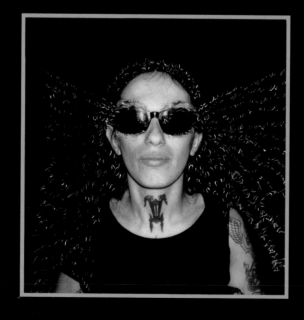

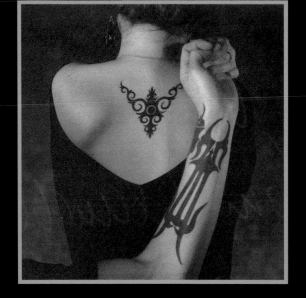

Dedication . . . for Pierrette

Acknowledgements

Big thanks to the following people who generously contributed to
this book:-
Mr Loubet, Mark Thackara, Phil Morley, Ian McDonald, Lisa and Lisa, Lionel
Tichener, Pete Trew, Steff Murschetz, Lisa and Kevin, Kaisu and David,
Anne, Alex Binnie, Spider Webb, Nakano, Chuck, Sammy Streckenbach, Lal Hardy,
Ian of Reading, Steve Beard, Eva and Gerry, Keith and Chris,
Erik Reime, Teena, Mickey Sharpz, Skin Deep Tattoo, Maui and Honolulu,
Jane Nemhauser, Tim Coleman.

Special thanks to Olympus Optical, UK and Germany; Tattoo Clothing
Paris, Geneva and Dusseldorf; Satellite Labs, London; Trew Photographic,
London, North America Travel, Sussex, England; Ilford Photo, UK; Fuji UK;
Scale Reprographic, London.

Equipment and materials used:
Olympus OM2N, Zuiko Lenses, T32 and T8 Ringflash,
Ektachrome and Fuji Velvia handline processing at The Lab, Tel. 071 250
1471; Ilford HP5 Plus, processed at Trew Photographic, Tel. 071 253 1600,
London

Other titles by Chris Wroblewski:
Modern Primitives
Skin Shows: The Art of Tattoo
Skin Shows II: The Art of Tattoo

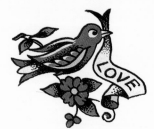

The Tattooed Lady: a Mythology

by Steve Beard

Antonia Gibson was a farm girl from Wisconsin, who, at the age of fourteen, ran away from home to see the world. Little did she know how things would work out. Once she had bumped into Charles 'Red' Gibbons, it was the world which travelled to see her. It started innocently enough, with 'Red' tattooing a cute little angel on her wrist. And maybe it ended innocently too. By the time Antonia finished her career as a tattooed lady with the Ringling Bros, and Barnum and Bailey freak shows, the only part of her not tattooed below the neck was her posterior. When fully clothed, she appeared so prim that most people mistook her for a retired school teacher.

Furthermore, the designs this staunch Baptist chose to adorn her body with were eminently respectable. Not only was there a portrait of the baby Jesus on her left thigh and a Madonna on her right, but there was a version of Botticelli's 'Annunciation' on her left arm, Raphael's 'Angels' below her left shoulder, and Michelangelo's 'Holy Family' on her biceps. Just in case anyone was unsure of her patriotism, there was a portrait of George Washington proudly emblazoned between her breasts.

Showing off her tattoos at the carnival allowed her to make a good living. Antonia was just one of a whole tribe of tattooed men and women who flourished in the fairs and carnivals of America at the turn of the century. In 1890, the first tattooed lady, La Belle Irene, appeared. She was similarly covered from head to toe in tattoos. Among the butterflies, flowers, angels and sentimental vignettes, her body was also decorated with such sanctimonious inscriptions as 'Nothing without labour' and 'Never despair'. She set a trend. This habit of draping scrolls of words across a background scenography of hearts and flowers came to be seen as typically American.

Also typical was the way in which La Belle Irene not only made a spectacle of her own body, but managed to extract a narrative from it as well. She told the awed punters who flocked to gawk at her that she had been tattooed way out West, in an effort to escape the sexual attentions of the Red Indians who still roamed there, tattooed savages to a man. It was a complete fabrication - but that was the point. This was

a woman attempting to negotiate for herself the cultural terms in which her naked body should be publicly addressed. Tales of forced abduction and desperate seduction - including all the stock elements of the escape-from-a-fate-worse-than-death school of narrative - were from then a regular feature of any tattooed lady performance at a freak show.

What both these case histories reveal is how a whole complex of diverse cultural issues can be condensed into a single, highly memorable figure. There is the aesthetic issue. Antonia's painted flesh not only bore tribute to the masterpieces of Renaissance culture, it also attempted to establish its own claims to be taken seriously as an expressive art, rather than just another dumb carnival turn. In that sense, Antonia and La Belle Irene may be seen as naive precursors of the self-conscious exponents of body art so visible in the post-Warhol Sixties and Seventies. Here was art liberated from the confines of the gallery and taken to the heart of Middle America. Here was a new folk art displayed proudly on the backs of the people. Here was an end to self-appointed experts and the culture of the museum.

Related to this is the religious or, in its broadest sense, the sacred dimension of the tattooed body. Antonia's tattoos may have taken their inspiration from the Renaissance masters, but they were primarily an index of her devotion to the Good Lord. The unconscious impulse at work in this respect was sacrificial. Antonia was both the executor and victim of a symbolic rite which, by denuding, penetrating and anointing her body, sought to prepare it in advance for the heavenly kingdom. The act of tattooing her flesh with images drawn from the Holy Bible transformed it from a profane icon into a sacred text. In a repetition of the original divine act, it made the Word flesh.

There is also something highly sexual about the sight of a pierced and striped female body. Without getting lost in the thickets of Freudian scholarship, it is possible to conceive of the tattooed lady as a brilliant fetish object, a symbolic phallus standing in for the real thing, which is typically so undependable, so shrivelled by the fear of failure and cancellation. Castration, that nightmare scenario of the

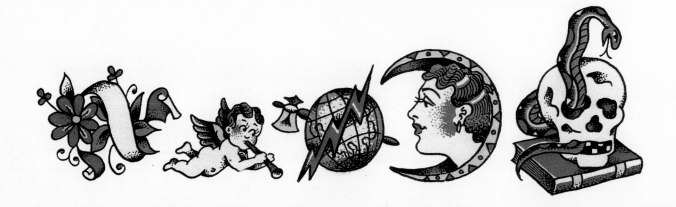

average screwed-up male, is a spectre which the fetish object evokes only to exorcise - it is played with, paraded, stroked, parodied. With a figure like Antonia or La Belle Irene, the body of the erect woman is mutilated and then venerated in a gesture of perverse eroticism. The sexual charge is indirect and works essentially as a form of narcissism. There is no coyness here. The appeal of the tattooed lady lies in her indifference.

Then, there is the issue of the body as social property. The tattooed lady exists on the border between public and private, abnormal and acceptable, visible and concealed. Here, the bare fact of its adornment translates the body into a freakshow pathology, a crowd-pleasing spectacle and a profitable commodity all at the same time. This is immediately complicated, of course, by the fact that the body in question is female. Antonia changed her name from Gibson to Gibbons at the same time as she was put to work in the carnival. The pictures her husband carved into her flesh were badges of ownership and advertised items of craftsmanship as much as anything else. When Antonia submitted to the needle, it was not only her flesh which was pricked; the very letters of her name were rubbed out and rearranged.

Whether considered in aesthetic, religious, sexual, or social terms, the tattoo is first and foremost an inscription, the primitive writing of power. It records the submission of the individual body to a collective code. No wonder La Belle Irene felt compelled to come up with her story of wild Red Indians and mutilation-under-protest. The tattoos on her body were the visible mark of her subjection to an alien law, an unknown imperative menacing in its imaginary fury. She needed to emphasise her status as a victim in order to restore an innocent blush to her skin; only then could respectable folk not feel unnerved at the sight of her. Her story was a fabrication, but it remained ambiguous, poised between claims of civilised behaviour and intimations of savagery.

This brings into focus the whole history of interaction between Europe and the New World. Ideological constructs such as 'savagery' and 'primitivism' emerged as a function of the colonial impulse, and served to legitimise acts of wholesale slaughter. The stories of forcible tattooing, which became popular at carnivals after the closure of the frontier, were cultural fantasies disguising what had been repressed, the brute act of genocide. It was the American native who had been displaced by the European settlers; the savages who had been exterminated by the civilised. The tattoos displayed on the bodies of carnival exhibits and freak show performers bore mute witness to this fact. History is writing before it is speech.

How old is the tattooing habit? Some have traced it back to the times of flint, soot and cave painting. Others have speculated that when there was the body, there was the mark. For evidence of the oldest tattooed lady, it is necessary to go back 4000 years, to the eleventh dynasty of ancient Egypt. When the mummified body of a priestess of the goddess Hathor was discovered at the site of Thebes, it was observed that she was tattooed with a pattern of dots and dashes on her lower abdomen, thighs and arms. Her name was Amunet. Egyptologists have hypothesised that these marks would have performed double duty, as the sign of both carnal appetite in the here-and-now, and lofty ambition in the hereafter. It all added up to a good resurrection.

Before Christianity got a grip on the world, tattooing was a common tribal custom. It was practised by the Ancient Picts and Celts of the British Isles, by the Ainu of Southeast Asia and Japan, the native tribes of the Americas, and the Polynesians of the South Pacific (the tribes of Africa, owing to their different complexion, went in for scarification rather than tattooing). In all these cultures, tattooing belonged to a symbolic order of birth, copulation and death, which was celebrated and understood by all. There was no nonsense about personal expression here.

Things changed with the advent of Christianity. According to Biblical lore, the human body is made in God's image and it is therefore sacrilegious to disfigure it in any way. Tattooing was considered to be a gross act of blasphemy, a pagan custom which required stamping out. A sign of the times is provided by the 787 Council of Churches meeting at Calcuth in Northumberland, which explicitly forbade all forms of tattooing. Similar decrees were passed

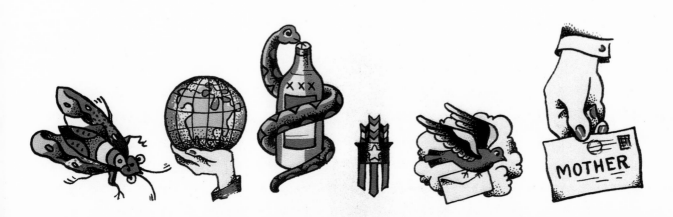

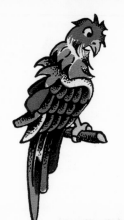

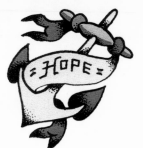
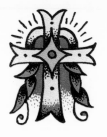
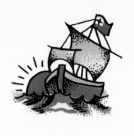

intermittently for the next thousand years. It was not until sea-farers and explorers of Christian Europe came into contact with the peoples of Asia, Africa and the Americas in the sixteenth and seventeenth centuries that the custom was reintroduced.

For the early colonists and explorers, tattooing seemed a charming novelty. A certain John Smith who visited the New World in 1593 recorded of the native inhabitants that 'some have their legs, hands, breasts and faces cunningly embroidered with diverse marks, such as beasts and serpents artificially wrought into their flesh with black spots', while in 1632 one John Bulwer wrote of the practice thus: 'About their legs strange lists they there doe make, Pricking the same with Needles, then they take Indelible tincture: which rub'd in, the Gallants doe account their bravest gin.'

It was the voyage of James Cook to the South Sea Islands, however, which was responsible for imprinting the custom on the public consciousness. Not only did he bring back a tattooed Polynesian, named Omai, to London in 1774, and display him all over town before returning him to his native island, but he popularised the use of the word itself, which was derived from the Tahitian 'tatau', meaning 'to mark'. In his journals, he describes with enthusiasm the circles and crescents, the human figures, dogs and birds which are recurring motifs in Polynesian iconography. And he is knowledgeable about the procedure involved: 'They stain their bodies by indentings, or pricking the skin with small in-struments made of bone, cut into short teeth; which indentings they fill up with dark blue or blacking mixture prepared from the smoke of an oily nut.'

When Cook took Omai to London, the Polynesian islander was a sensation. Back home, though, he would have been just another member of the tribe. This expresses the difference between the tattoo perceived as an aesthetic spectacle, and the tattoo recognised as a tribal mark, and neatly encapsulates the continuing split between the functional and purely expressive uses of the custom. For someone like Omai, tattooing was a way of life. It was the ceremony attached to successive rites of passage: entry into the tribe, access to manhood, entry into marriage, passage into war, journey into death.

As for the tattooed ladies of the tribe, the celebrated rite was likely to be initiation into puberty. The anthropological data reveals just how much the practice of tattooing women functioned as a form of pricing and branding in the marriage market. The *Ainu* tribeswomen, for example, were tattooed on the lips at birth, and on the arms, once they were be-trothed or married. The job might have been done by the women of the family, but it was clear it was meant to benefit the husbands and fathers of the tribe. For a young tribes-woman from Port Moresby, meanwhile, things were even simpler. The more tattoos she had, the more suitors she could expect, and the higher her price. With a system like this in place, it was not long before girls were being tattooed from head to foot, even on the most sensitive areas of the body like the insides of the thighs.

The first tribesperson to be exhibited in London was a tattooed lady. After Martin Frobisher returned from one of his voyages to find the North West Passage in 1578 he brought back an Eskimo woman and paraded her through the capital. Contemporary drawings reveal that she was tattooed with blue-black lines of dots which curved gracefully along her cheeks, chin and forehead. James Burbage had opened the first Elizabethan playhouse only two years earlier, and it is likely that the Eskimo woman took her place alongside the barbarian Turks, depraved Jews and monstrous kings of the stage as one more painted devil.

At the same time, the sight of her scarred face would not have been that unfamiliar to an Elizabethan audience. Just as popular as the exotic marvels of the stage in early modern England were the bloody spectacles of the scaffold. Here, condemned men were ritually cut open and tortured prior to their execution in coded ceremonies of power, which paid symbolic tribute to the king or queen of the day. According to the French historian Michel Foucault, such events were essentially episodes of sovereign inscription, where the law of the land was carved directly into the bodies of those who had themselves violated it. Despite the sanctimonious edict of the Council of Churches meeting at Calcuth, it seemed that some bodies were less valued than others.

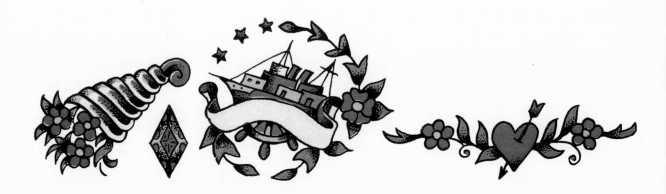

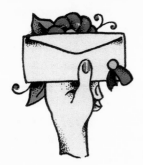  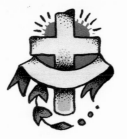 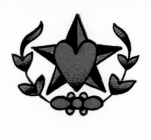

In succeeding centuries, according to Foucault, the state developed less spectacular ways of making its presence known to those who wronged it, at the same time as it transformed the category of primary offence from treason to deviation from the social norm. A new species of public enemy was created - the delinquent rather than the traitor - whose body was still subjected to the force of the law but was no longer directly marked by it. Instead of being brutally attacked, it was slowly worn down by the punishing grind of exercises and examinations, which was the daily routine of such 'carceral' institutions as the prison and the barracks.

All very humane. And a much more efficient method of social control. Cultural theorist Michel de Certeau observed the history of changing technologies of bodily restraint, or of 'writing machines': 'In order for the law to be written on bodies, an apparatus is required that can mediate the relation between the former and the latter. From the instruments of scarification, tattooing, and primitive initiation to those of penal justice, tools work on the body. Formerly the tool was a flint knife or a needle. Today the instruments range from the policeman's billyclub to handcuffs, and the box reserved for the accused in the courtroom.'

What both Foucault and de Certeau fail to notice, however, is the persistence of an older technology of inscribing power within carceral society. Tattooing, far from being 'primitive', remained an instrument of social control up until fairly recently. It was not until 1879, for example, that the British Army stopped tattooing deserters with the letter 'D' and men of bad character with the letters 'BC'. Meanwhile, inmates of Siberian prison camps and Nazi concentration camps have been tattooed with identifying signs or numbers in ways which still haunt society today. Even the stalwart matrons of the Salvation Army were, properly considered, tattooed ladies, given that they had the initials of their organisation tattooed above their elbows.

But even this is not the whole story. For soldiers, sailors and prisoners were also in the habit of tattooing themselves. Anchors, flags, shields, skulls, hearts, crucifixes, serpents and naked ladies: a whole panoply of signs appeared like a semiotic rash on the bodies of the incarcerated, on their

backs and arms and chests and legs. Here was a reminder of another law quite different from that of the state. It was thus no surprise that towards the end of the nineteenth century a body of ethnographic and anthropological literature was produced whose stated aim was the decipherment of this perplexing phenomenon.

In 1881, for example, a certain Dr A Lacassagne published the results of his survey of 1333 tattoo designs, taken from 378 men of the 2nd Battalion in North Africa. He classified them into seven groups: patriotic and religious, professional, inscriptions, military, metaphors, amorous and erotic, and fantastical and historical. To the good doctor this riot of signs must have seemed like evidence of a regression to savagery on the part of those it decorated. With the benefit of hindsight, it can be seen as something quite different: an act of ritual reversal and symbolic defiance, a protest against the degrading conditions of carceral society made by its inhabitants from the material of their own bodies.

The spread of this practice can be put down to the invention of a 'writing machine' not mentioned by de Certeau: the electric tattooing needle. Patented by Tom Riley in 1891, this device effectively put an end to the older technique of hand tattooing, and tattooing parlours employing it soon sprang up in most ports and industrial cities. By the middle part of the present century, this new technological development had been joined by the mass production of pattern charts to make the whole process cheap, instant and efficient. New designs appeared which were influenced by the early mass media, and it was not unusual to see strapping men sporting portraits of cinema characters like Tom Mix, Felix the Cat or Mickey Mouse on their arms.

Tattooing, however, was by no means an activity confined to the depths of society. In the very early years of the century, a fashion developed for unusual and intricately wrought tattoos among the hooligan rich. Famous politicians, tycoons, entertainers and aristocrats paid astronomical fees to have various designs emblazoned on the most conspicuous parts of their bodies. Such insinuating sexual motifs as butterflies and spider's webs were popular with women, and it is here that the tattooed lady reappears in different guise, as a

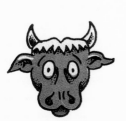 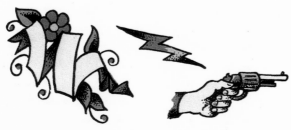 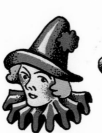 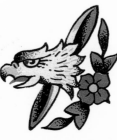

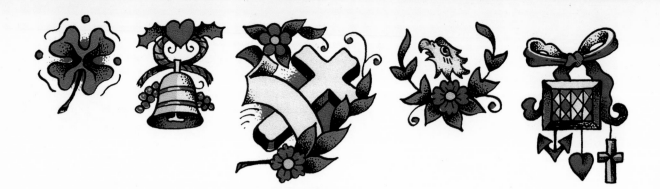

that the tattooed lady reappears in different guise, as a celebrity rather than a freak. Lady Randolph Churchill, for example, was one of the first tattooed ladies of the smart set and had the image of a serpent eating its tail tattooed on to her arm as a symbol of eternity.

There was also a brief fad for cosmetic tattooing, which involved society ladies being faintly tattooed on their cheeks and lips in order to improve their complexions. Some even went as far as having their eyebrows and eyelashes tattooed. The whole ritual generally took place in a plush clinic and was heavily invested with an atmosphere of grave deliberation and surgical precision which meant that the word 'tattooing' was never mentioned. As George Burchett, celebrity tattooist to the Mayfair crowd, comments in his memoirs: ' We boasted a staff of lady assistants, dressed in the sombre uniforms of hospital nurses, and one invaluable asset, a well-educated and finely spoken receptionist, who received instructions to inquire "very, very discreetly" the patient's name.'

Under this combined aspect, the tattoo functioned no longer as either a badge of belonging or a mark of protest but as a fashion statement. Like all fashions, its tenure was brief. The commercialisation of tattooing soon identified it in the public mind as a nasty proletarian habit and society ladies were soon much less willing to submit themselves to the attentions of a shifty man with a needle. By the Twenties, Lady Randolph Churchill had taken to hiding her tattoo beneath a bracelet, while the whole business of cosmetic tattooing was no longer anything to boast of. There must have been many fashionable women who would have blushed at the memory of their past indiscretions, if only they were able to.

It was not until the postwar years that tattooing was again to come into vogue, partly as a result of the dialectic between mainstream and marginal forms of behaviour sparked by the hippy and punk cultures. Both, in their different ways, contributed to a revival of body conscious-ness, a reclamation of conventional signs of exclusion and a redefinition of notions of primitivism. Equally important to the increasing respectability of the custom, however, was the

fact that the tattooists themselves had cleaned up their act. No longer operating out of shady backstreets, they sold themselves as artists and behaved like professionals. They sterilised their equipment, charged by the hour rather than by the piece, and inclined towards customised work rather than standardised designs.

Add this all together and you come up with what some have deemed a tattoo Renaissance. According to this symbology, tattoos are no longer so much social markings or even fashion statements, as they are high-minded instances of body art. As such, they can range from traditional Japanese detail work covering large areas of the body, to black graphic tribal insignia snaking down an arm or a leg. The conventional iconography of hearts and flowers, meanwhile, is written off as an example of the 'international folk style', an idiom which, according to the critic Marcia Tucker, is characterised by 'agglomerate designs, often executed by many different tattooists on a single client, which results in a "collection" of conflicting styles, sizes and images.'

It seems that even in the world of tattooing there is a hierarchy of taste. It is one which women, in particular, are entirely familiar with. One conspicuous feature of the tattoo renaissance is the number of women, often highly educated and with powerful careers, who wish to decorate their bodies. A consultation with their tattooist, for these post-feminist creatures, has all the secret excitement and cool deliberation conventionally associated with a visit to the mall. Here is an American tattooist's description of one such client: ' A chick came in to get a tattoo yesterday. She was really serious about it. She brought in all these books, and we spent over an hour deciding on the design and where it should go. She was really artistic herself. She finally decided on a stylised Indian bird design on the side of her breast.'

This new class of self-empowered tattooed ladies is something explored by Chris Wroblewski's photographic portraits in the following pages. What soon becomes clear is that there is something very postmodern about this phenome-non. The wealth of anthropological and ethnographic information made available in recent years, the explosion of

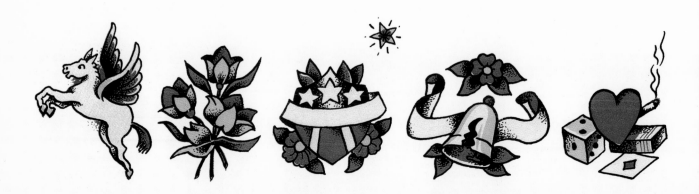

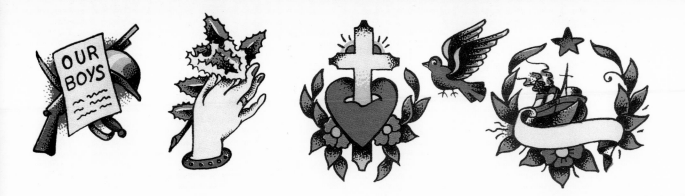

mass media imagery, the increased visibility of graffiti and other forms of street rhetoric, the fascination with the iconography of other cultures - all have played their part in developing a repertory of images which the prospective client is able to sample at her leisure when choosing a tattoo. As the scholar Arnold Rubin puts it, she is free to adopt 'the marks of a Maori chief, a North African courtesan, a pirate, an Indonesian headhunter, a Japanese samurai, an outlaw motorcyclist, a Scythian warrior, a Buddhist monk or a twenty-first century time traveller'.

It would be easy to conclude from this seductive litany that the tattoo has completely lost its subversive charge, its power to shock and revivify. Cher would be the central figure in this argument. The internationally renowned rock star and actress has had almost as many tattoos as she has surgical nips and tucks, and seems to feel that they are as equally cosmetic. According to this way of looking at things the tattooing needle would then take its place alongside the surgical scalpel and the benchpress as one more medically-boosted 'writing machine'.

But that would be to underestimate the irrational power of the tattoo, its continuing psychological efficacy as charm or magic amulet. This is something else in which Wroblewski is clearly interested. A previous collection of his portraits of tattooed figures was published under the title *City Indians*. It neatly sums up the idea that once traditional ceremonies of incorporation lose their power, people begin to work out their own personal rites of passage directly on their bodies. What is finally suggested by Wroblewski's work is a less celebratory phrasing of the postmodern condition than the one conjured by the tattoo renaissance, a condition marked by crisis, doubt, confusion and perhaps the dream of a resolution in a New Tribalism, a global collective which cuts across differences of race, class and gender.

According to this dispensation, the tattooed body is no longer treated in aesthetic terms as a blank canvas awaiting the ministrations of the divinely inspired artist, but is considered instead as a *tabula rasa* overlaid by the hastily scribbled hand of experience. The tattoo recovers its meaning as a mnemonic device, a way of tying a knot in the

flesh, of recording a moment of love, a departure or arrival, a pilgrimage, an insult, a birth or a death. It is a message from the present to the future self. In that sense it gives a new value to the muddled collage of inscriptions so deplored by the celebrants of the tattoo renaissance, and reveals the buried life beneath the dead phrase 'international folk style'.

At its purest, the tattoo is not an aesthetic, religious, sexual or social event. It is a ritual engagement with death. This is the real meaning of Cher's tattoos. Like her subjection to the surgeon's scalpel, her submission to the tattooist's needle represents an attempt to arrest the ageing process, except now conceived in magical terms as a spell cast on the surface of the skin, designed to prevent its inevitable deterioration. As a postmodern tattooed lady, Cher cuts a more elaborate figure than that of Antonia Gibbons - but not a less human one.

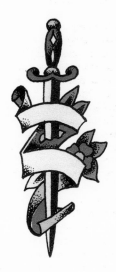

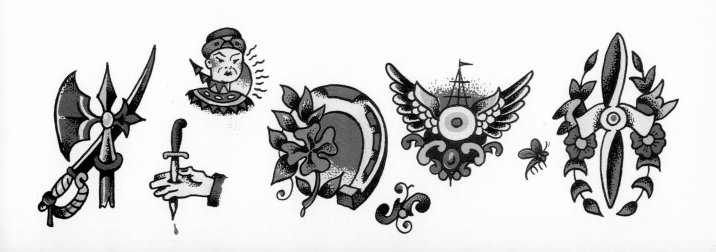

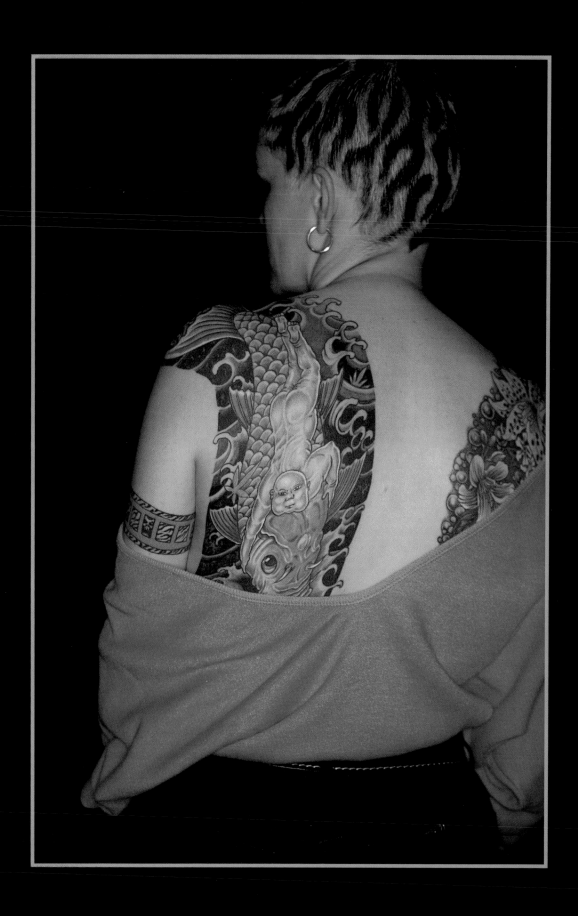

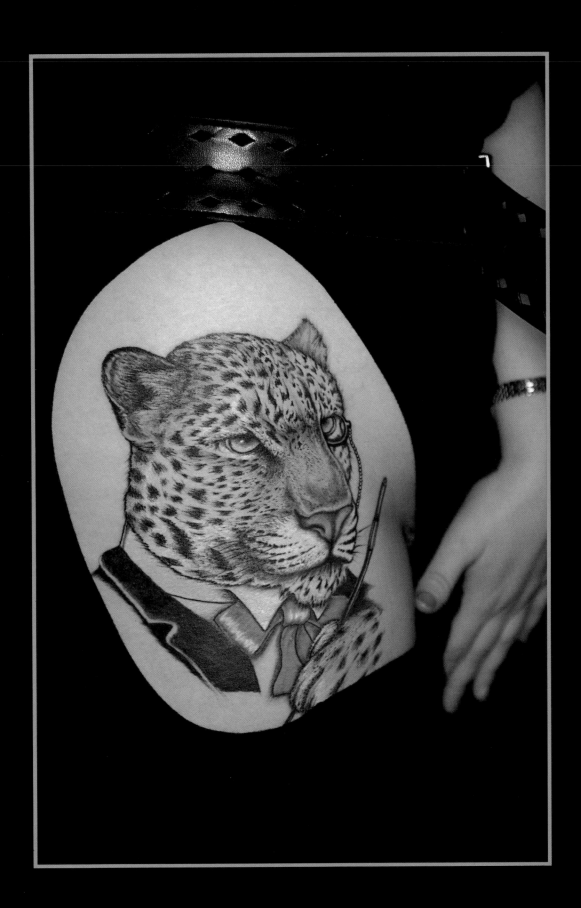

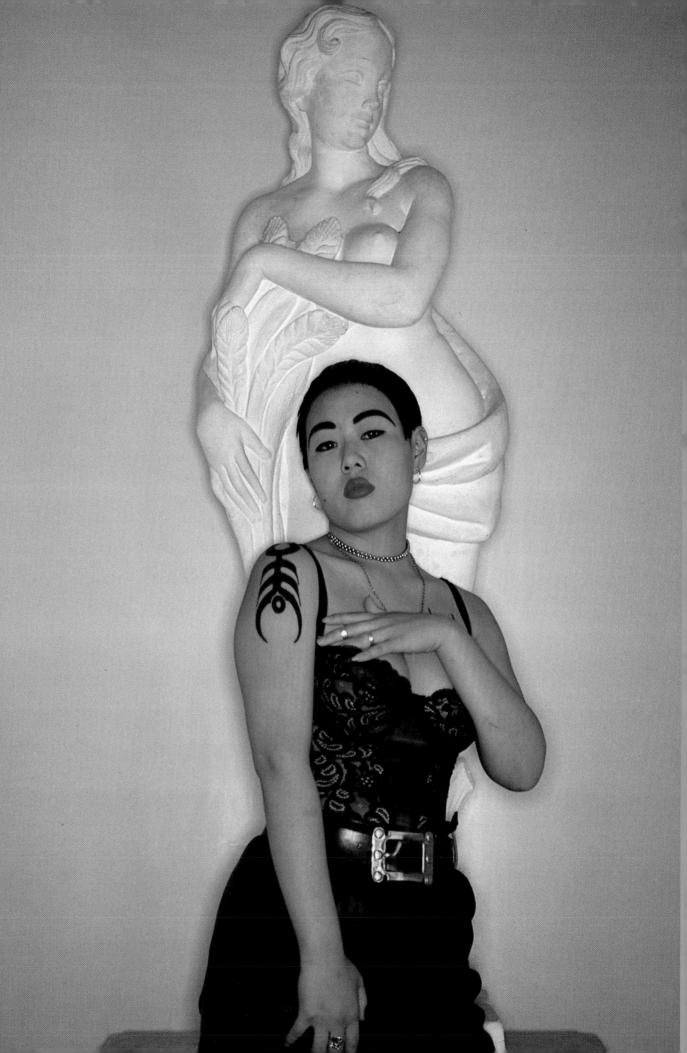

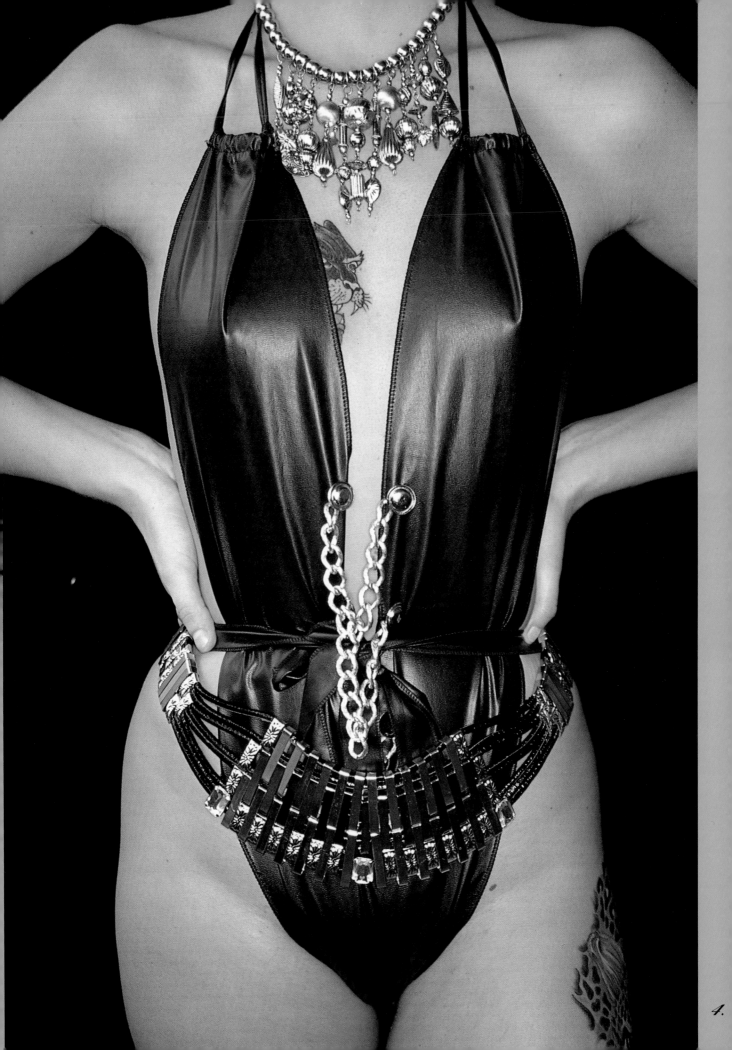

4.

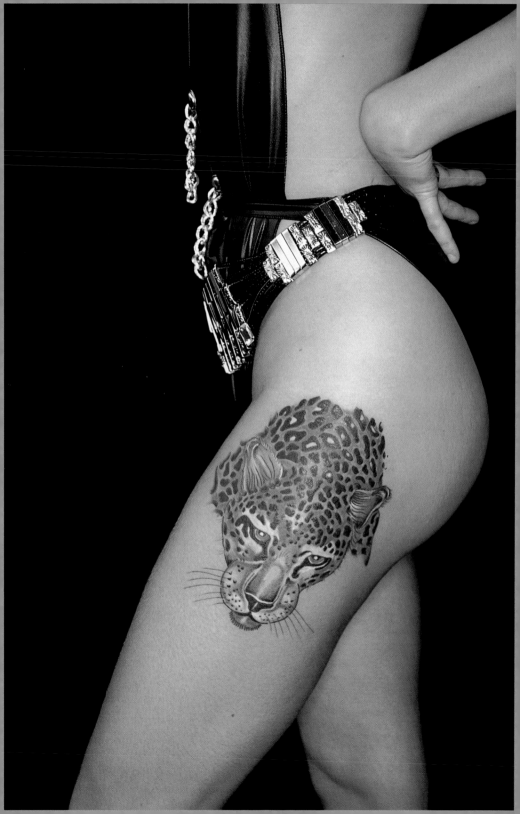

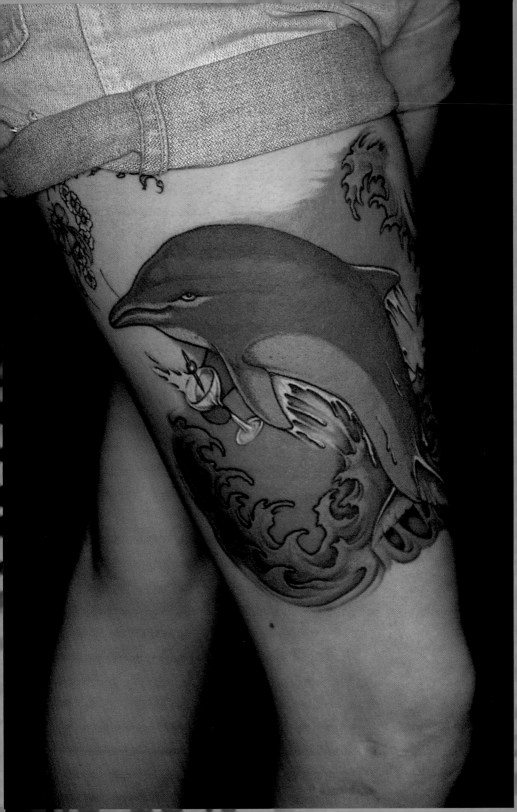

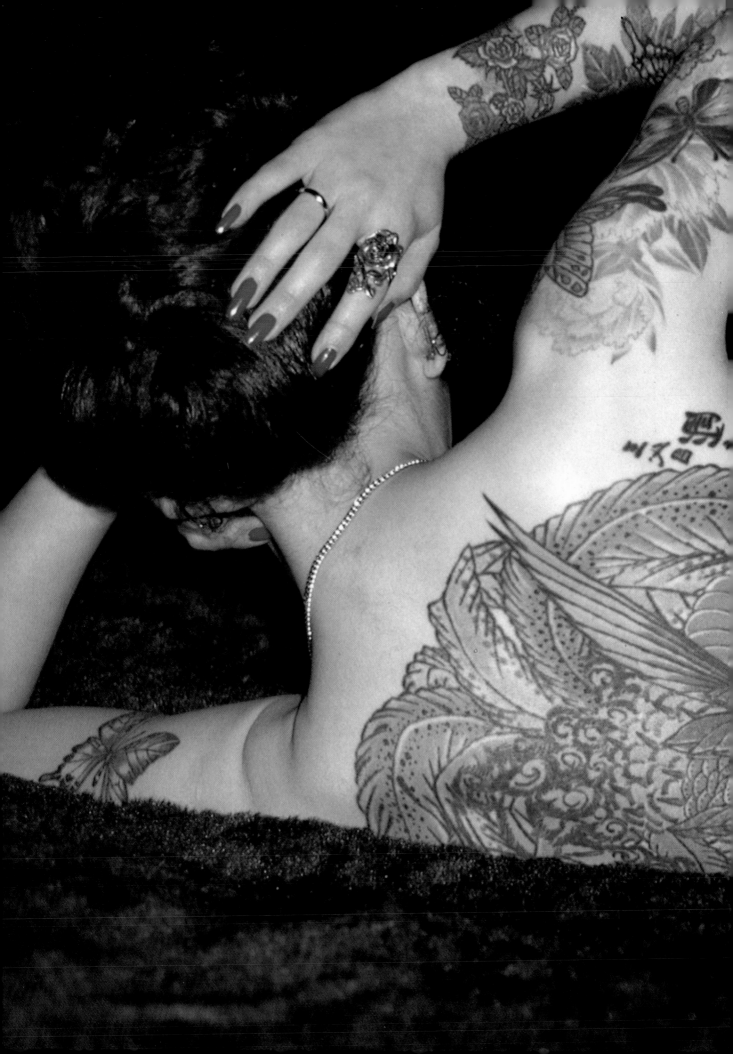

In the Ryu-Kyu islands of Japan, many tribes practised tattooing, and it was common for women to have their forearms and the backs of their hands marked with indigo patterns, which identified her family. The legends tell that a nobleman wanted to carry off a Ryu-Kyu princess. In order to put him off, she had her arms and hands secretly tattooed with a purple pigment, which convinced people that she had contracted a skin disease. The nobleman gave up his plan, and soon after tattooing became popular with the island women.

Girls from the Ainu people were tattooed on the mouth soon after birth, and the process completed when they were betrothed or married with the tattooing of their arms. It is said that this custom is derived from ancient times, when captive women were tattooed in order to show that they were the personal property of their captors. Unlike the Japanese method of tattooing (pricking the skin), the Ainu cut the flesh with a knife and then rubbed in wood ash. Perhaps the finished tattoo may be compared to the Western wedding ring, or the blackened teeth of a married woman in feudal Japan, signifying she was Taboo. This process was carried out by the girl's grandmother or her maternal aunt, who would tattoo the girl in three stages, each time broadening and darkening the design.

First the girl's lips would be washed with a solution of boiled birch bark, and the design would be outlined by cutting the skin with a flake of volcanic glass, or the point of a very thin knife. The blood was wiped away with a cloth, saturated in the solution, and then the soot from the birch bark would be rubbed into the wounds which produced a blue tint. In 1900 the Japanese outlawed this practice. However, the Japanese used several other characters to denote tattooing:-

Gei - an ancient word which denotes the blackening of the face, particularly around the eyes.

Irezumi - generally used on wrongdoers, and means to put ink into the skin.

Shi sei - an elegant term used to describe tattoos in general. It means to decorate the body with pictures or letters.

Horimono - describes artistic tattoos and means 'inscribed'.

Irebokuro - used in elegant language and signifies the making of a mark.

Gaman - means patience and self-control.

Aboriginal tribes such as the Ainu who tattooed their faces or shaded their eyes were described as having *gei*. During the Edo period after 1629, mistresses had the name of their lovers tattooed on their arms, or between their fingers. This was known as *Irebokuro*.

Yuki Desuos, wife of famous surrealist poet Robert Desuos (1900-45), had a siren on her leg tattooed by a famous painter, Foujita.

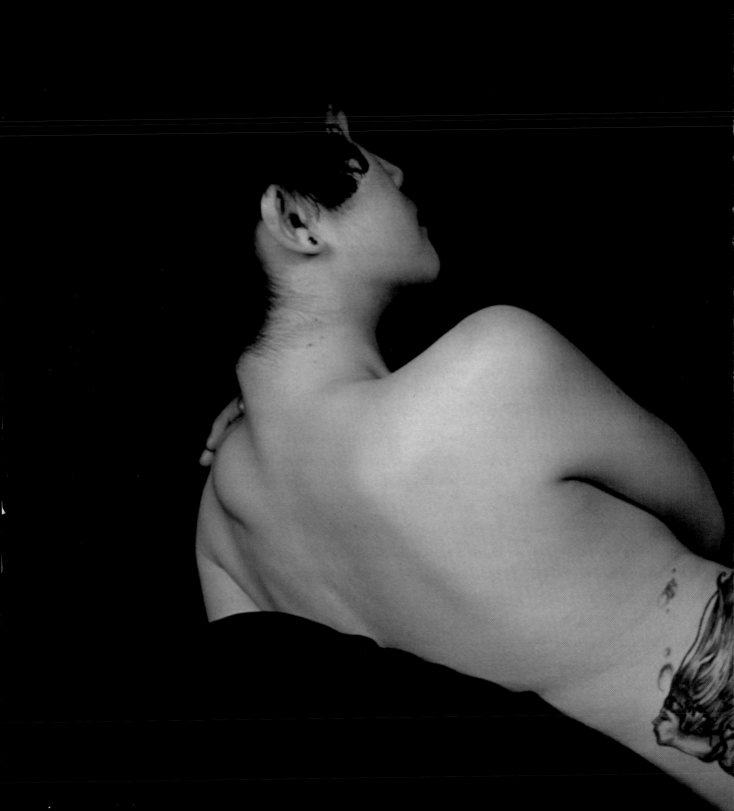

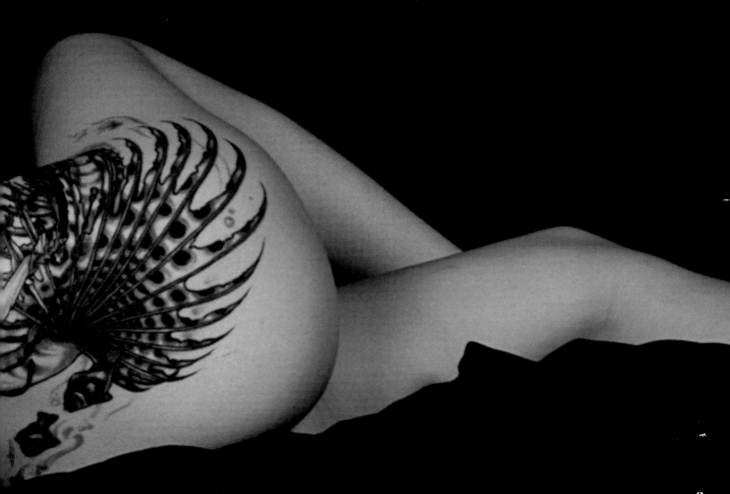

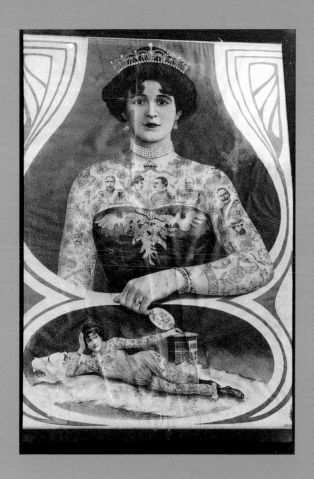

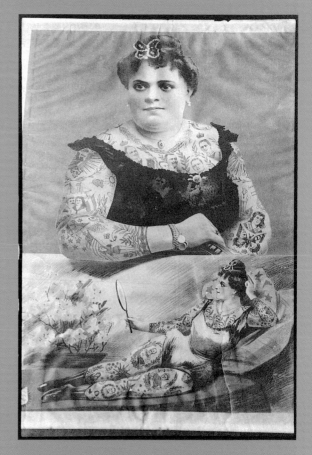

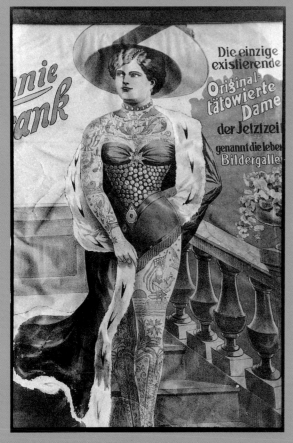

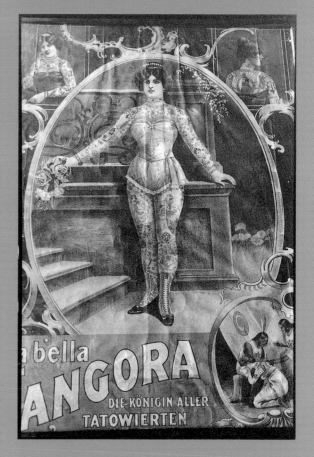

9.

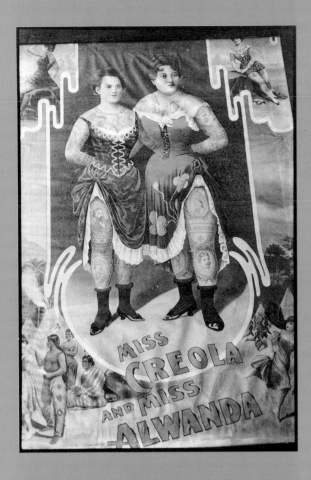

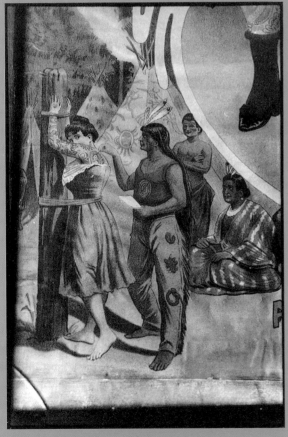

LA BELLA ANGORA was known as the Queen of tattooed people, and performed in Europe around the turn of the century. She sold picture postcards of herself after each performance in her lace boots, which were in fact tattooed on.

PRINCESS BEATRICE had the Last Supper tattooed on her back, which carried the admonition 'Do unto others as you would that they should do unto You'.

MRS BEN CORDAY was an English tattooed lady at the turn of the last century. A portrait of Queen Victoria was tattooed on her chest, topped by various coats of arms. On her right breast was written, 'Peace', and on her left breast was written 'Unity'. Her back was tattooed with a snake and two dragons.

DAINTY DOTTY, whose real name was Mrs Owen Jensen, was married to an L.A. tattoo artist. She worked as a fat lady with the Ringling Bros, and weighed 600lbs. She supposedly gave birth to a child in a tattoo studio without realising that she was pregnant. She worked as a tattooist in her husband's studio, and died in 1952 of a heart attack.

ANTONIA GIBBONS was born on a farm in Wisconsin in poverty. She only completed ninth grade at school and when she was fourteen she left to see the world. She met Charles 'Red' Gibbons at a carnival, who did a little angel on her left wrist as her first tattoo. She became married shortly afterwards and began her career as a tattooed lady with the Ringling Bros, Barnum, and Bailey freak shows. Except for her face and ass, she was tattooed up to her neck on every square inch of her body. She was a Baptist, and when dressed, everybody would take her for a retired teacher. Her tattoos consisted of a portrait of George Washington between her breasts, Botticelli's *Annunciation* on her left arm, Raphael's *Angels* below her left shoulder, and Michaelangelo's *Holy Family* on her biceps. On her left thigh was a portrait of the child Jesus, and on her right thigh, a portrait of the Madonna. On her right calf was Vermeers' *Diana and the Nymphs*.

LA BELLE IRENE was an American lady whose real name was Irene Woodward. She was the first completely tattooed lady to appear in Europe and was performing around 1890. Her body was covered with a multiple design of butterflies, flowers, angels and snakes. She was closely studied by the scientists of her time.

ANETTA NERONA was a German tattooed lady of exceptional talent, who worked around 1900, performing not only as a tattooed attraction but also as a magician, snake charmer and music virtuoso. Her body was tattooed with portraits of Goethe, Schiller, Bismark, Emperor Wilhelm II, and Richard Wagner.

LADY VIOLA was tattooed by Frank Gray, who placed the portraits of six US presidents on her chest and, a picture of the capital on her back. She dedicated her arms to the portraits of ten movie actresses and, her thighs and legs to Babe Ruth, Charlie Chaplin, Tom Mix and Captain Rosenthal.

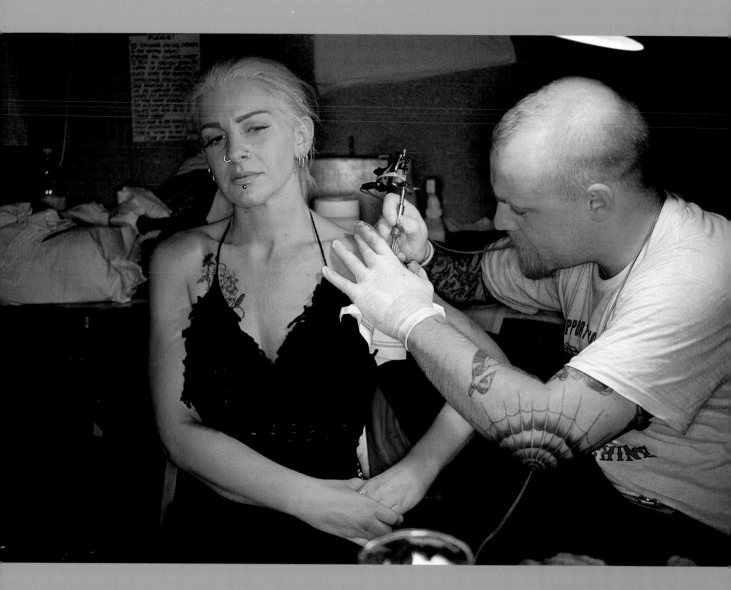

'Towards evening it grew cooler, and Tesse sat down on a flat stone at the edge of the tobacco patch. She was ready for the ordeal that would enhance her beauty.

The pain? The girls serenity denied all dread of it, and the presence of white skinned strangers, who would witness the cutting and scarring of her body, seemed not to ruffle her composure. Tesse already bore blisterlike scars from earlier cosmetic surgery. now she would receive three rows of cuts that would produce bumplike welts upon her left shoulder.

This additional stipple would allow Tesse to walk with new pride as a young lady almost grown up.

Kosse-Gogo, a woman skilled in these tribal rites, performed the surgical honours. Using a stout thorn, she lifted the skin on Tesse's left shoulder blade. Then, with the front edge of a small knife shaped like a spatula, she firmly made a short incision. Swiftly and deftly she repeated the process in a row of cuts. Blood trickled down but Tesse neither flinched nor showed any emotion'.

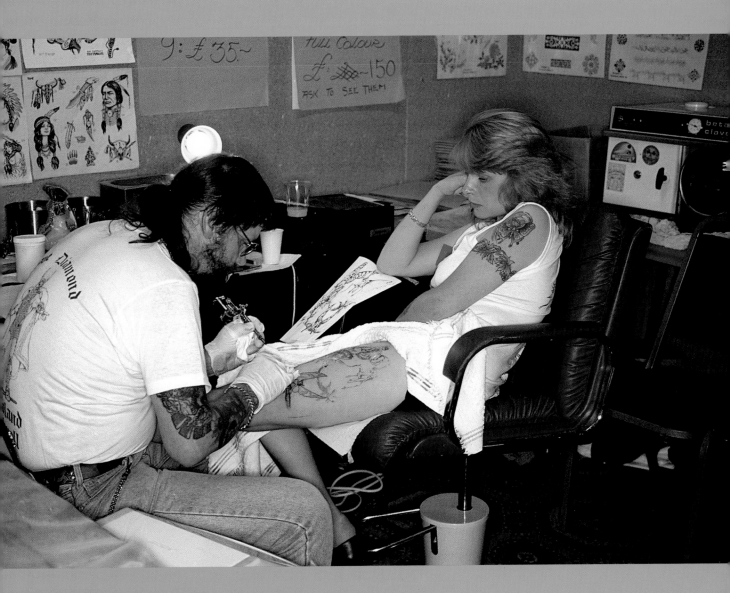

'Tattooing appears in the Middle Kingdom of Egypt and seems to have been borrowed from the Nubians' abstract patterns, which were composed of dots and dashes in a bluish-black colour. Tattooing was then regarded as one of several vehicles, by which the procreative powers of the deceased could be revived in the hereafter, in order to assure resurrection based on a complex Osarian model. The available evidence suggests that these women were associated with ritual music and, on occasion, with the Goddess Hathor'.

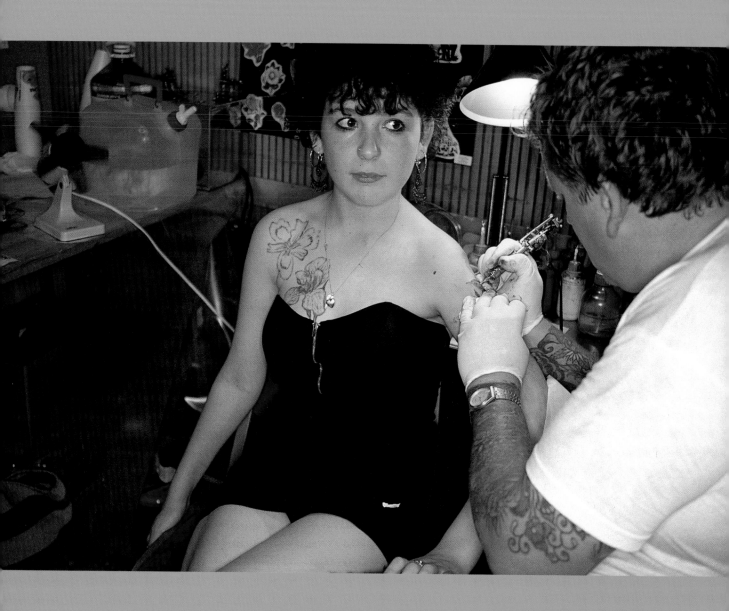

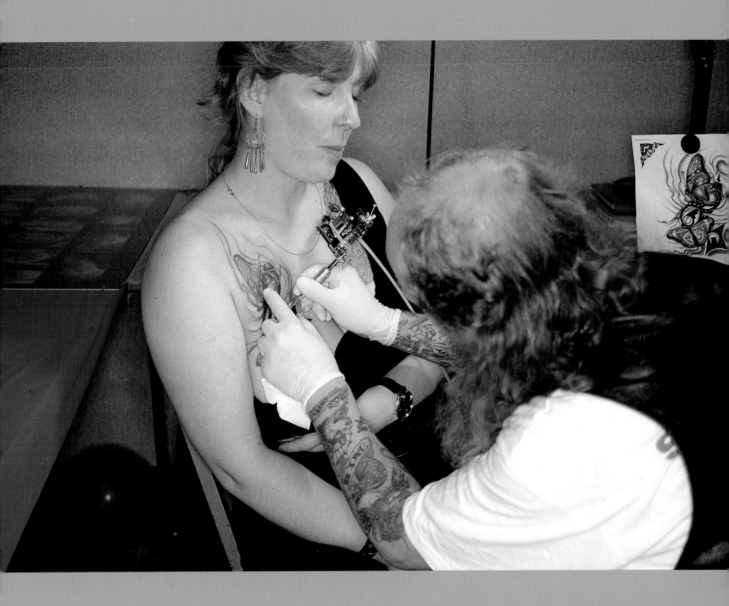

TATTOO GIRLS CHOOSE SUCH ODD SPOTS

Girls are going tattoo-crazy. They're flocking to tattooists to have names and pictures imprinted in the oddest places. Butterflies on their bosoms, boyfriends' portraits on their legs. Some even want to 'sit on' a tattooed reptile!

Top London tattooist Alexander Gordon said last night; 'I've had so many requests, I've had to leave my telephone receiver off. I've tattooed everything-yes-everything-from peacocks and stars' names to the signs of the zodiac'. And to prove it, he pointed to some photographs of recent jobs. There were housewives, typists, debutantes and models; with tattoos on their backs, thighs, stomach, everywhere ... Most popular with the debs, he said, are butterflies on the thigh. He did three in Mayfair last week. The average teenager likes the names of her pet pop singer or film star. One of Mr Gordon's young customers had Gregory Peck's name tattooed around her bosom twenty five times, with the names of all his films. There was only just room ... A Reading housewife got him to tattoo a butterfly on her tum, and a Red Indian on her chest. She hasn't got round to Davy Crockett yet.

In the provinces tastes vary. Leicestershire girls favour the American forces-names of boyfriends and Service insignia. Liverpool girls go for the names of sailors and their ships.

Don't sneer, men. Lots of you who have Marilyn Monroe on your mind, say the tattooists, have been getting her tattooed on your chest!

From an article in an English newspaper 1950s

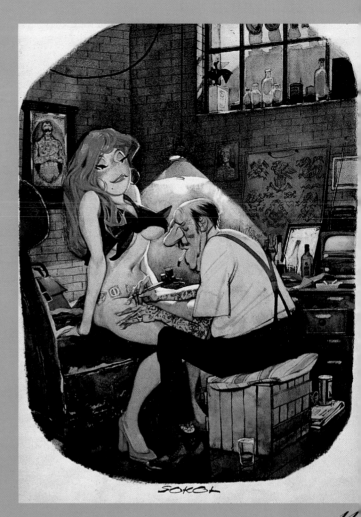

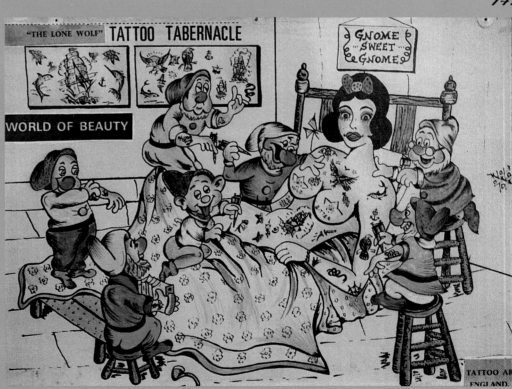

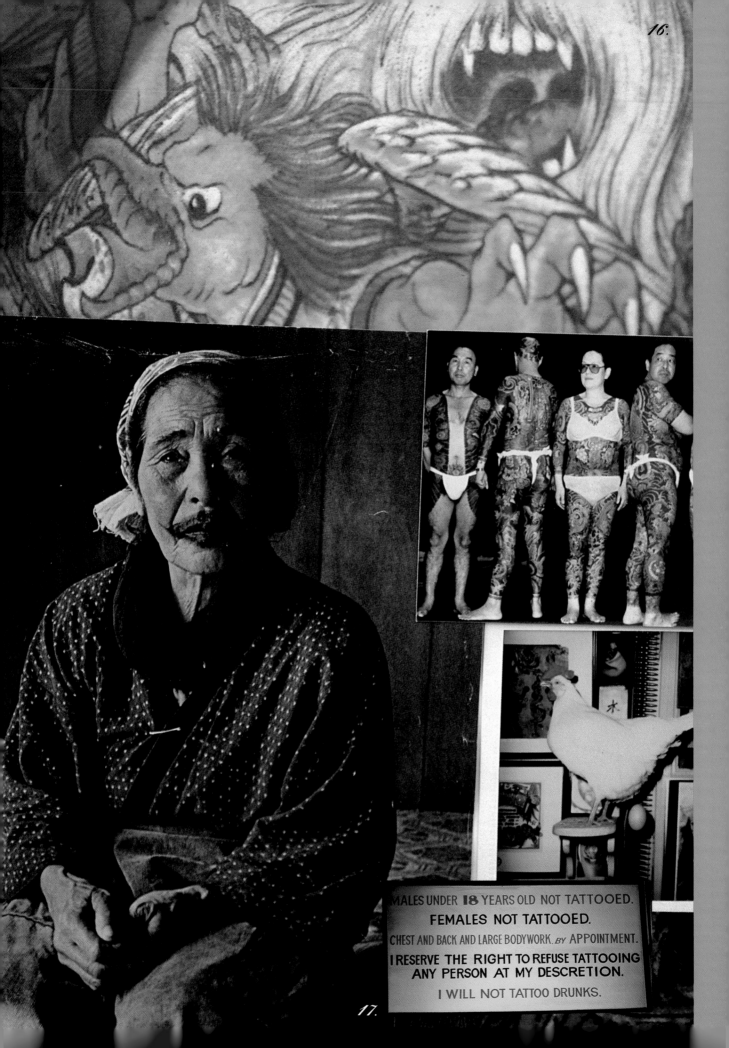

MALES UNDER **18** YEARS OLD NOT TATTOOED.
FEMALES NOT TATTOOED.
CHEST AND BACK AND LARGE BODYWORK. *BY* APPOINTMENT.
**I RESERVE THE RIGHT TO REFUSE TATTOOING
ANY PERSON AT MY DESCRETION.**
I WILL NOT TATTOO DRUNKS.

17.

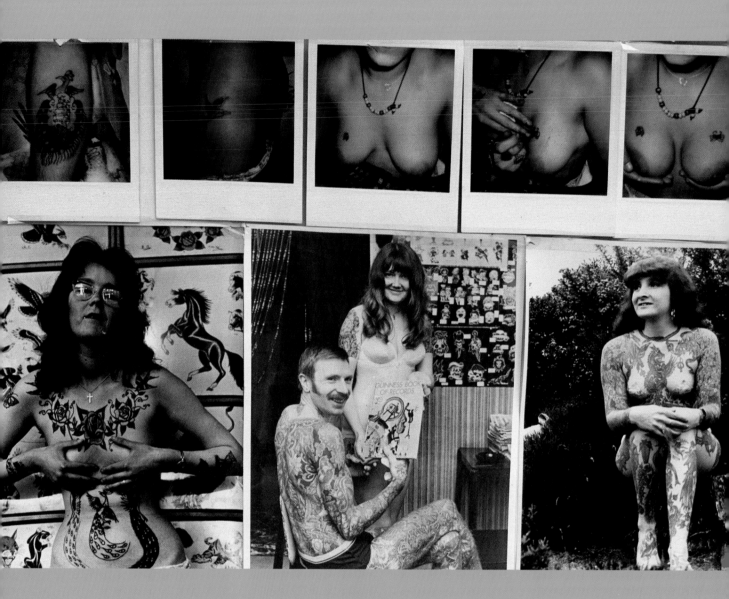

In January 1923, interest was suddenly diverted from the tomb of King Tutankhamen, to the discovery of a tattooed Egyptian princess in a tomb near Luxor. This royal lady was apparently one of the beauties of the first Theban dynasty which flourished more than 2000 years B.C.

Newspaper reports described her body as being mar- velously preserved, with the hair and teeth still intact. The body, slender and statuesque, had several dainty tattoo- marks, on one shoulder, the neck and bosom.

The reports added that the princess was probably one of the favourites of the Menthuhotep king, and that her narrow waist and slender hips suggested that such a figure was as much sought after by the ladies of Ancient Egypt as by modern women.

No sooner was the story printed, than I was besieged by ladies of all ages with orders for a 'dainty tattoo like the Egyptian princess's'.

George Burchett (1873-1953)

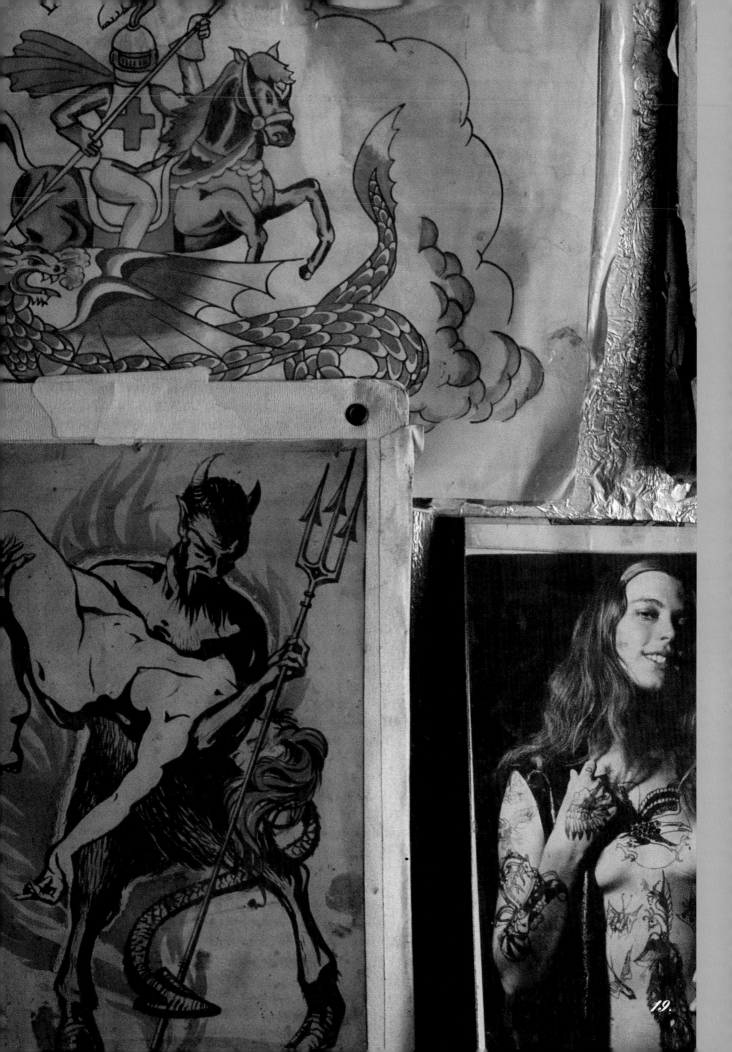

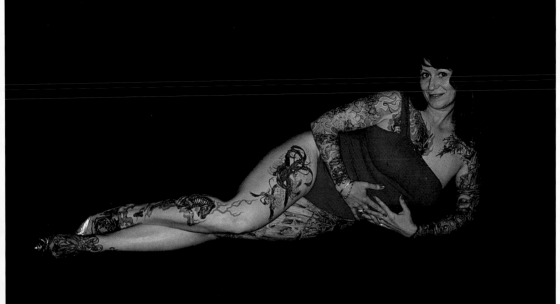
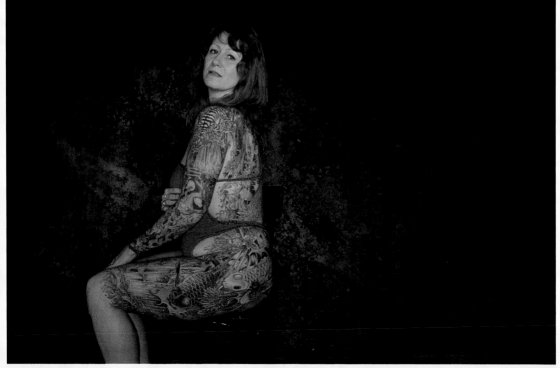

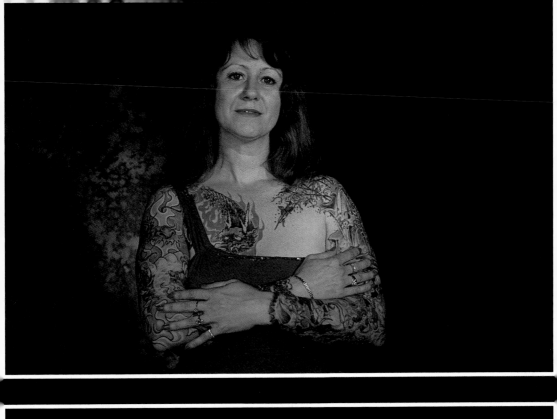
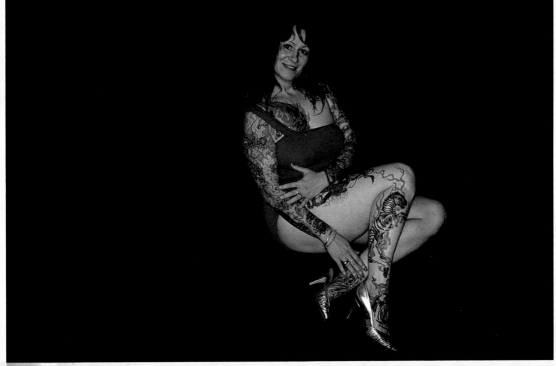

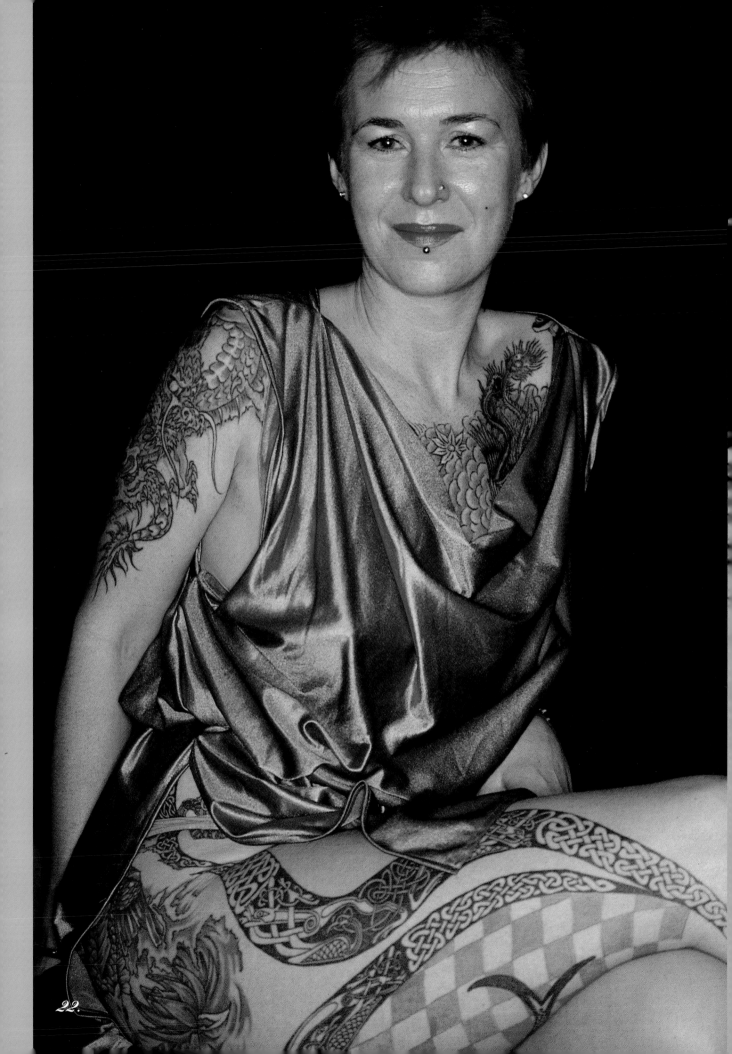

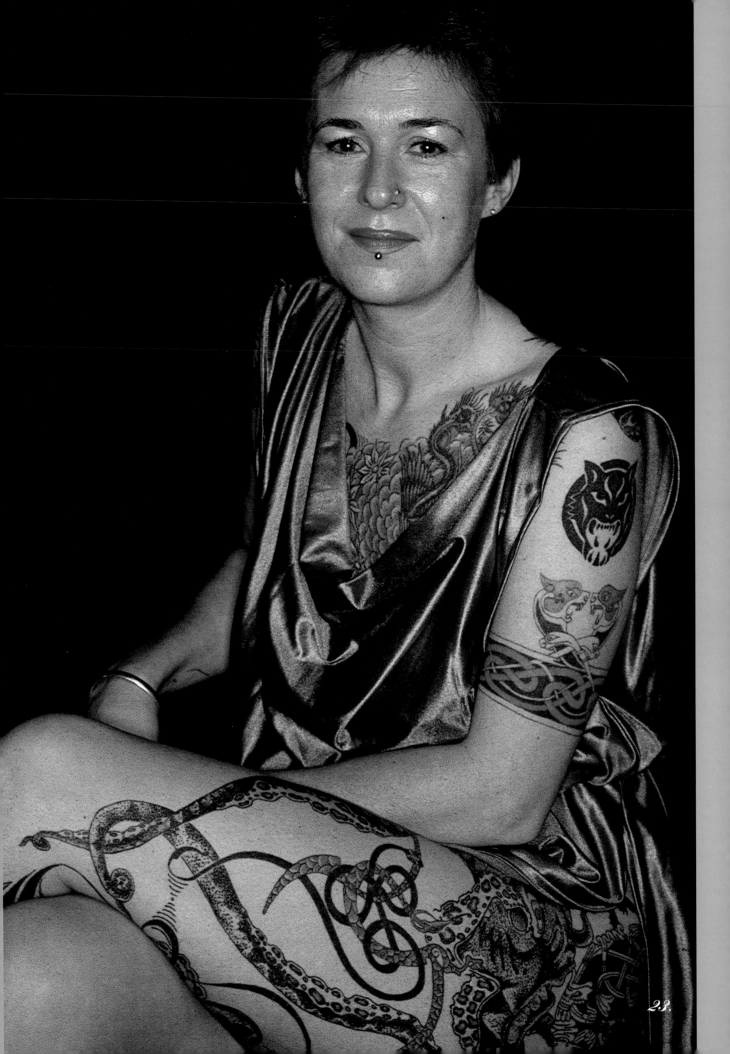

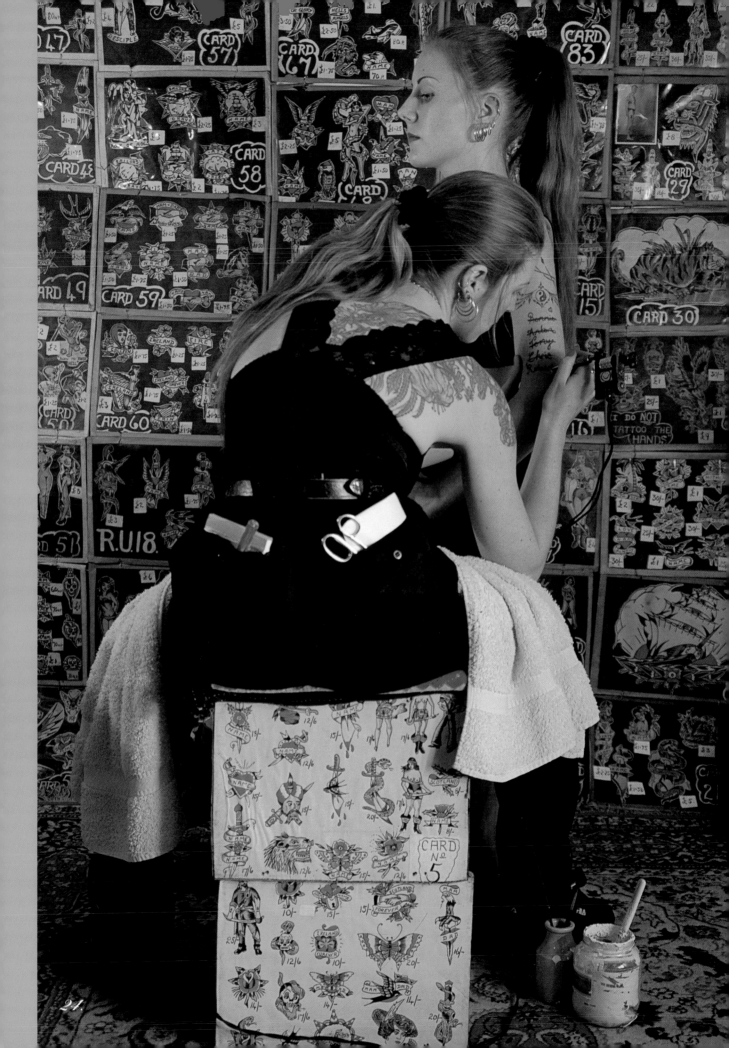

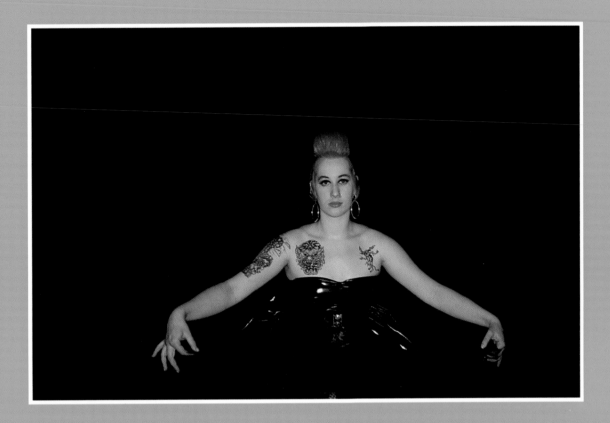

In 1578, the Arctic explorer, Sir Martin Frobisher, whilst attempting to find the North West Passage, came across an Eskimo woman, whose face bore delicate blue-black dots on her cheeks, chin and forehead. He decided to return with her and she was known to have been exhibited to a curious European public, thus setting a trend that would continue as long as the explorers and colonialists managed to find new cultures and ceremonies to plunder. At the Leipzig trade fair in 1899, twenty-three Samoan men and women were exhibited as an ethnographical item.

Meanwhile, Salome was busily attracting the crowds at fairgrounds and circuses throughout Europe in the last quarter of the 19th century.

She gave out a handbill that read:-

" Salome"
The only oriental beauty.
Tattooed in 14 colours.

The body of Salome represents a value
of 30,000 Marks and was a prizewinner
in Berlin, Vienna, Paris, London, New York,
St Petersburg ... 10.000 Marks reward
... pays Salome to the one who has seen
so much splendour of colour on anyone
else's body before.

On another stage in another country, Ubangi savages could be seen showing off their scarred faces and lip plugs.

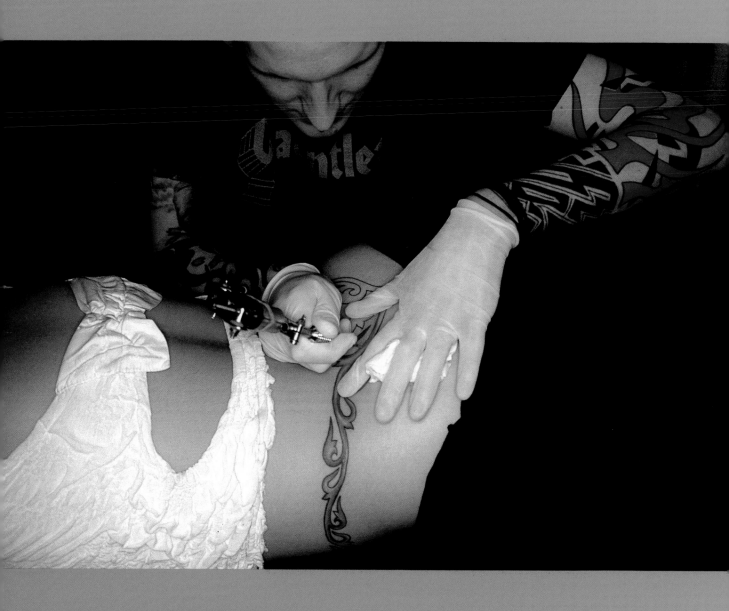

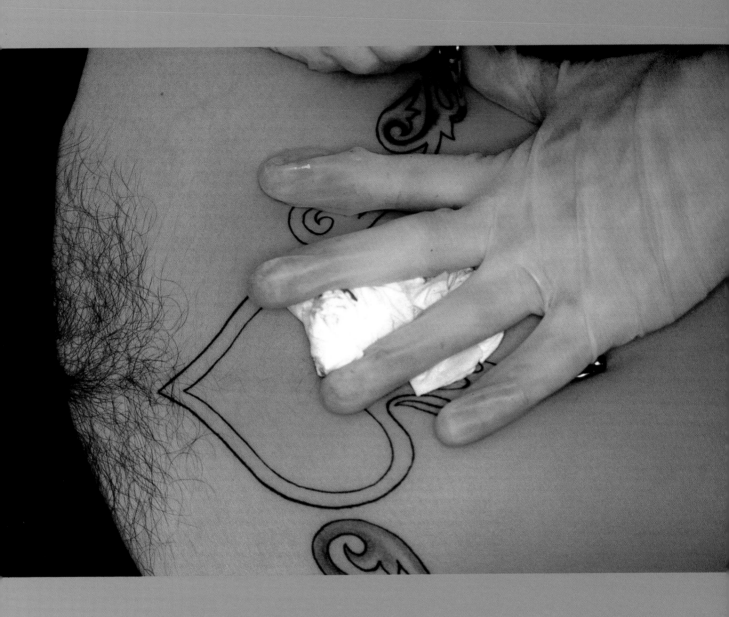

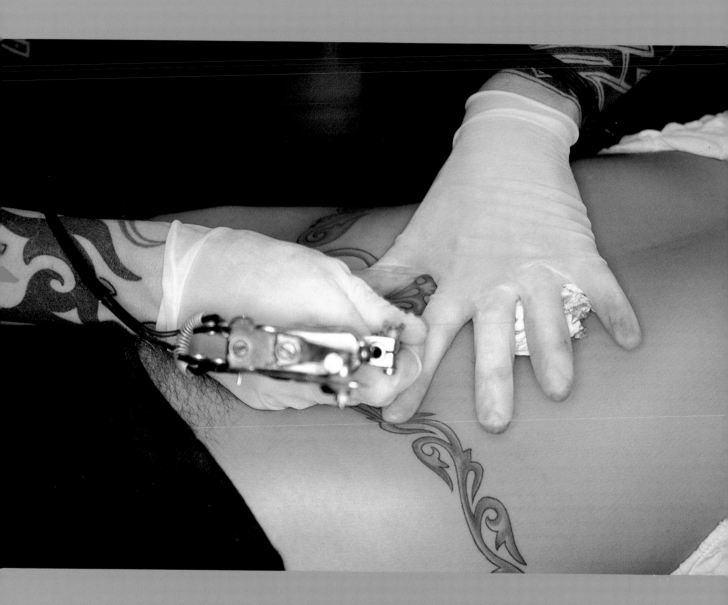

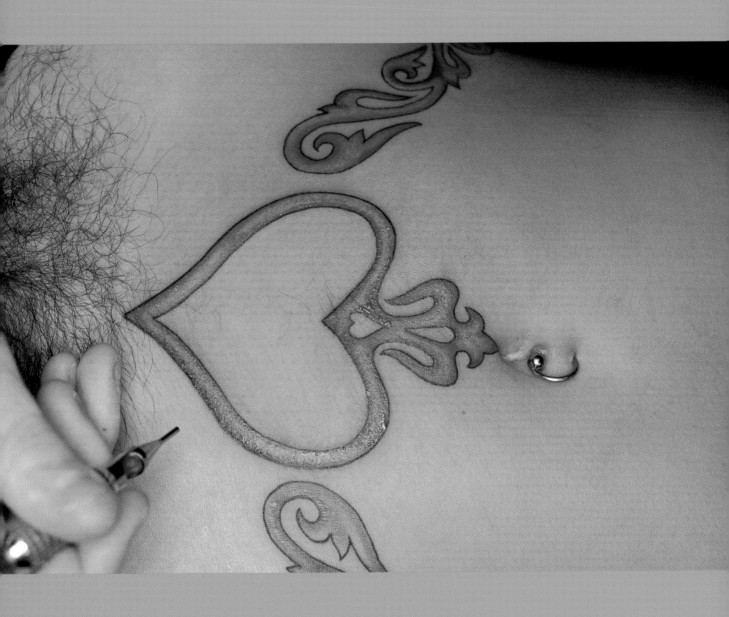

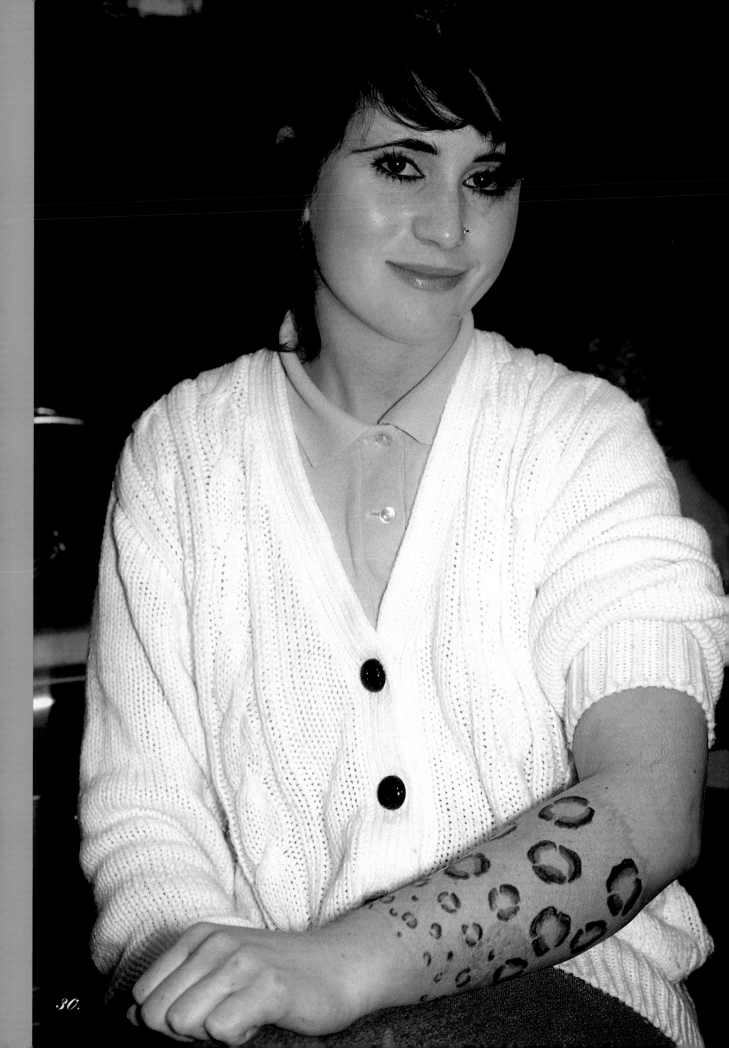

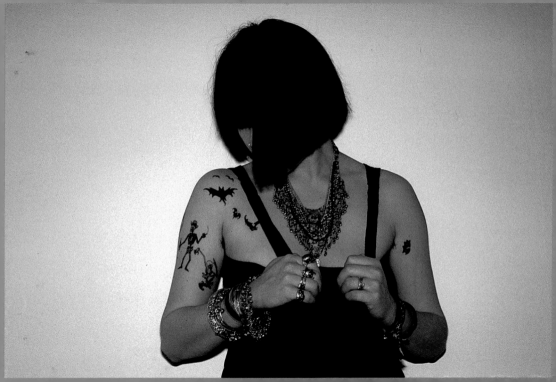

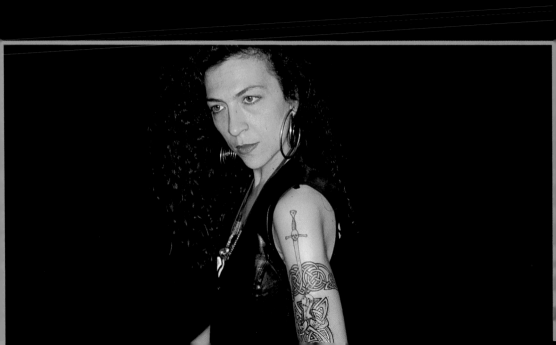

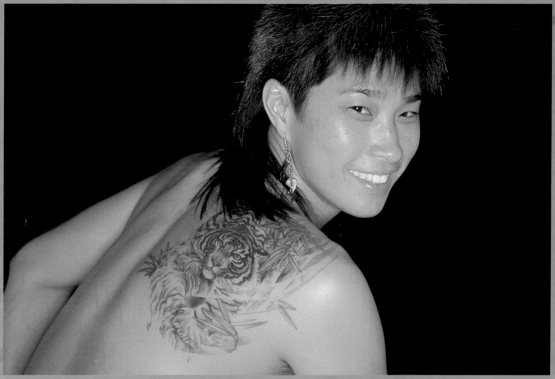

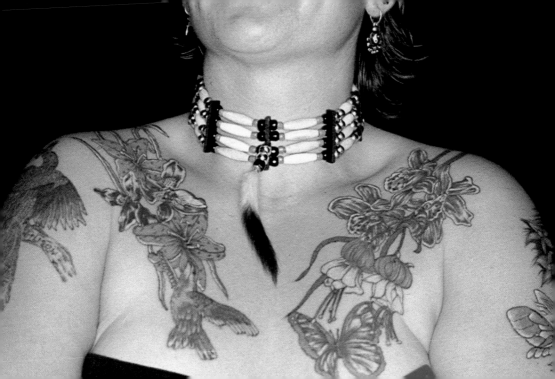

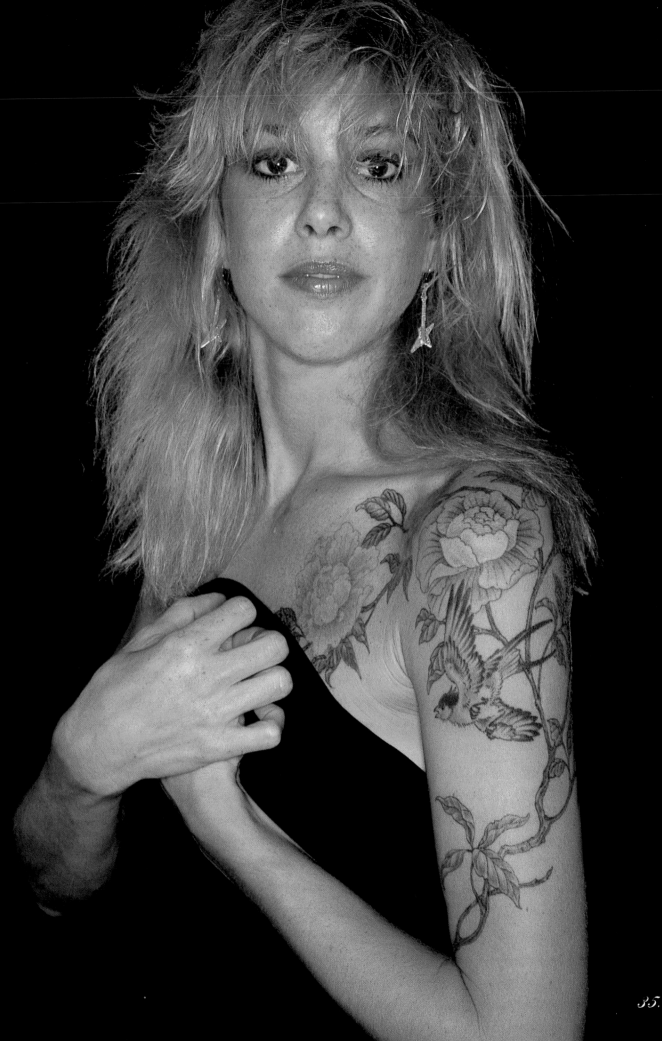

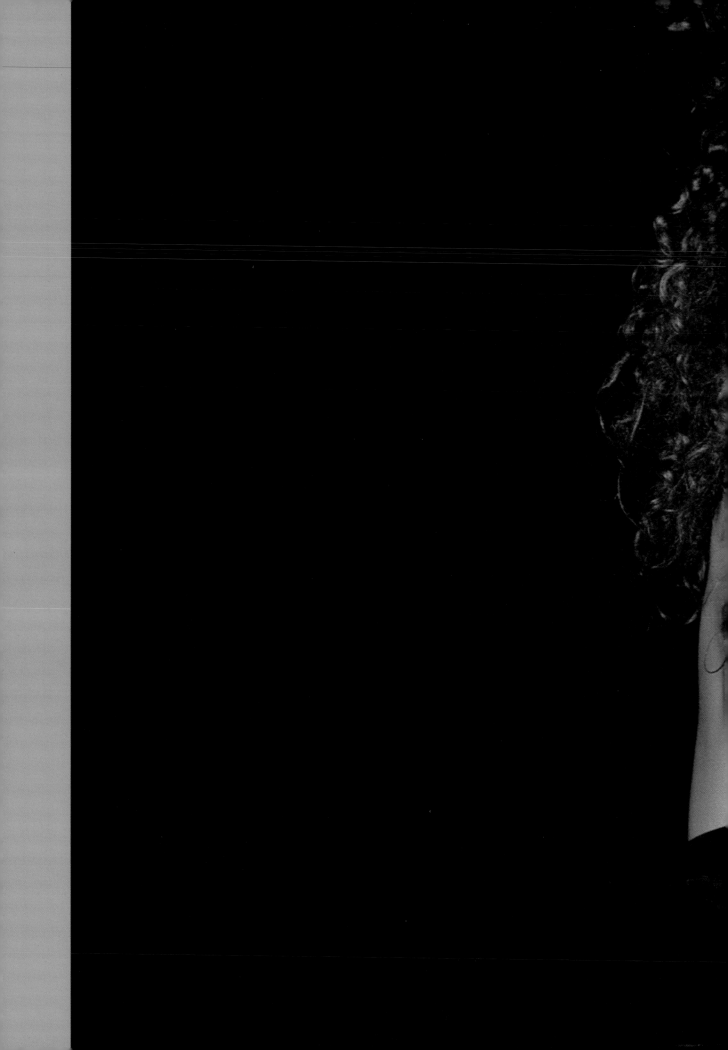

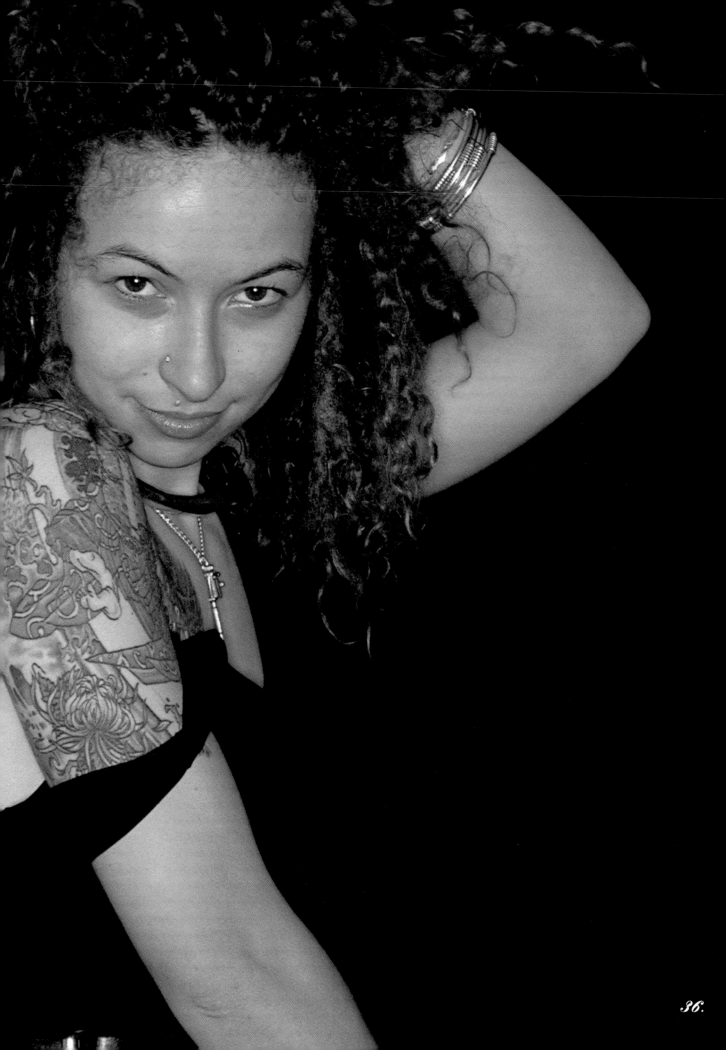

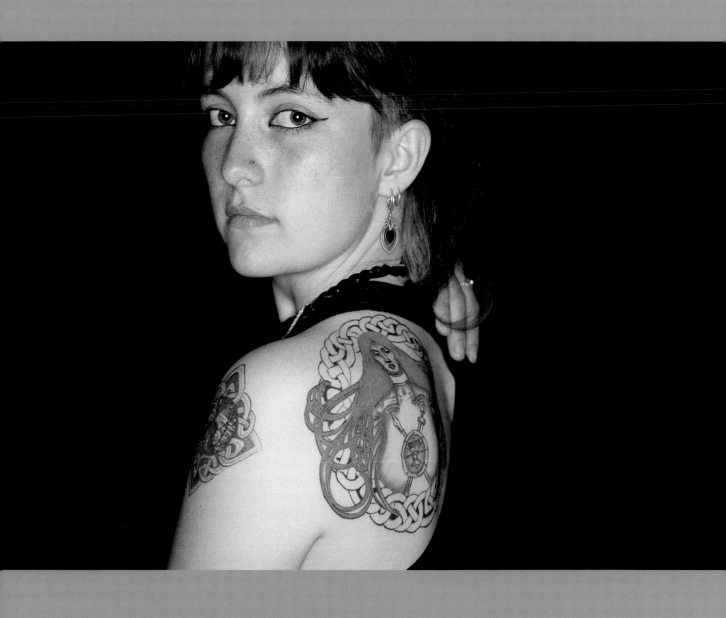

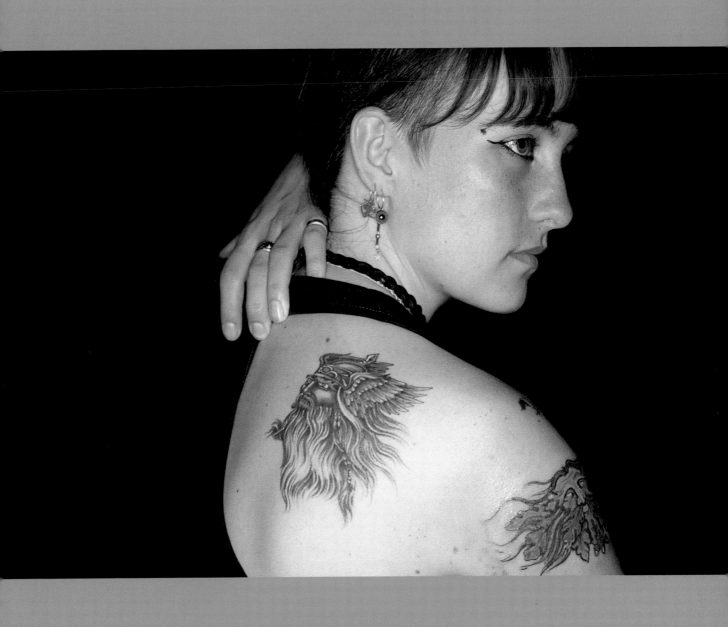

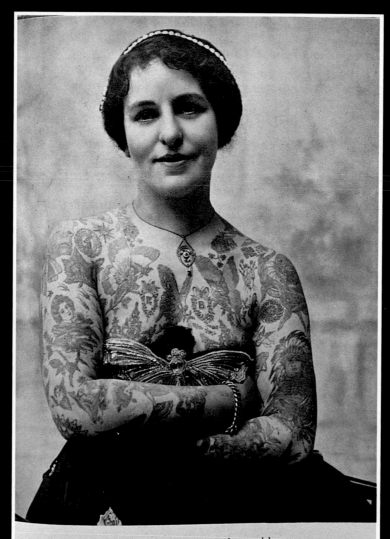

My dear wife, Edith, was my best model.

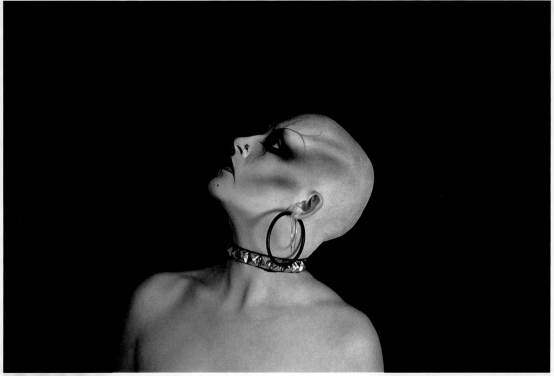

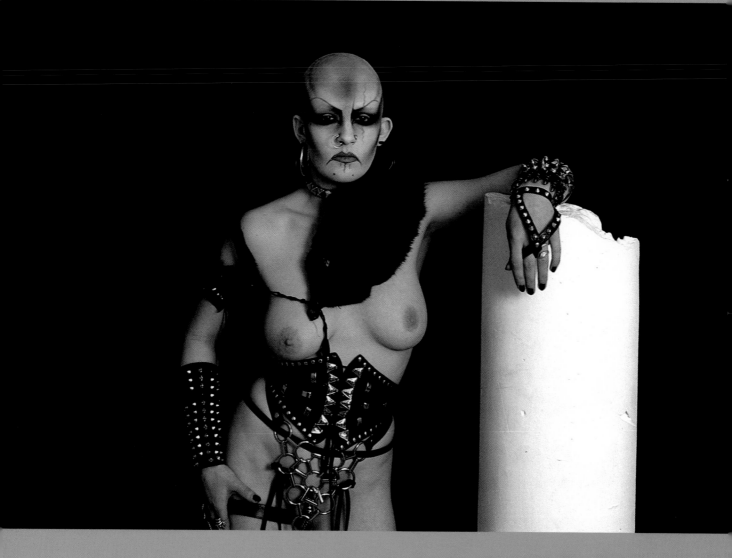

'Now I notice that some foreign peoples use certain plants on their persons both to make themselves more handsome and also to keep up traditional custom. At any rate among barbarian tribes the women stain the face using one plant and some other; and the men too among the Daci and the Sarmatae tattoo their own bodies. In Gaul there is a plant like the plantain, called glastum; with it the wives of the Britons, and their daughters-in-law, stain all the body and at certain religious ceremonies march along naked, with a colour resembling that of Ethiopians'.

From PLINY Book XXII

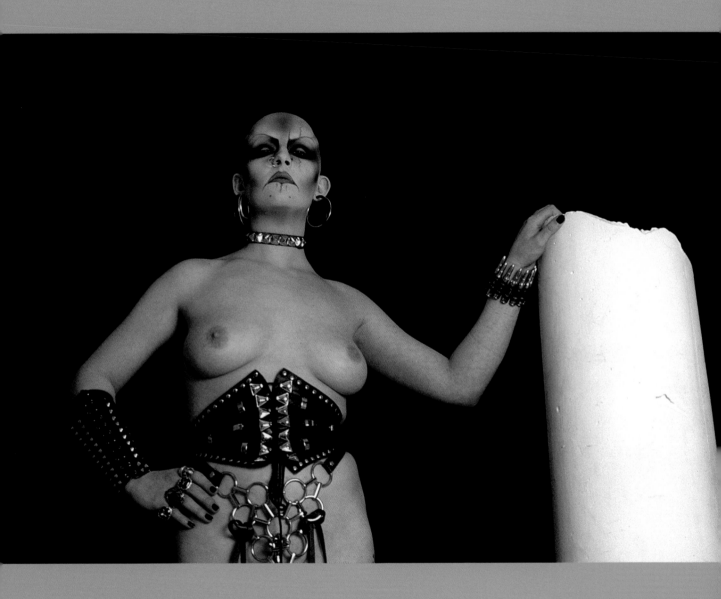

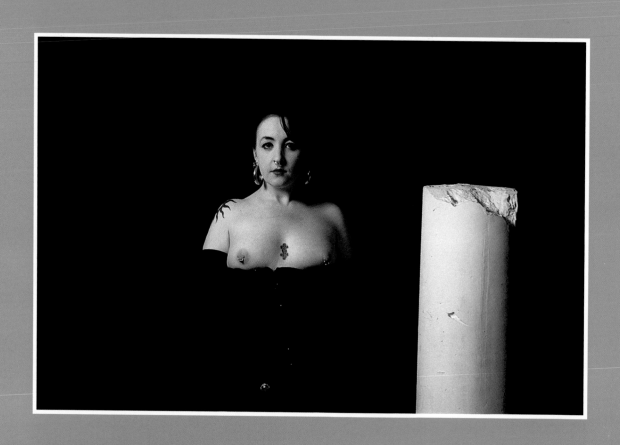

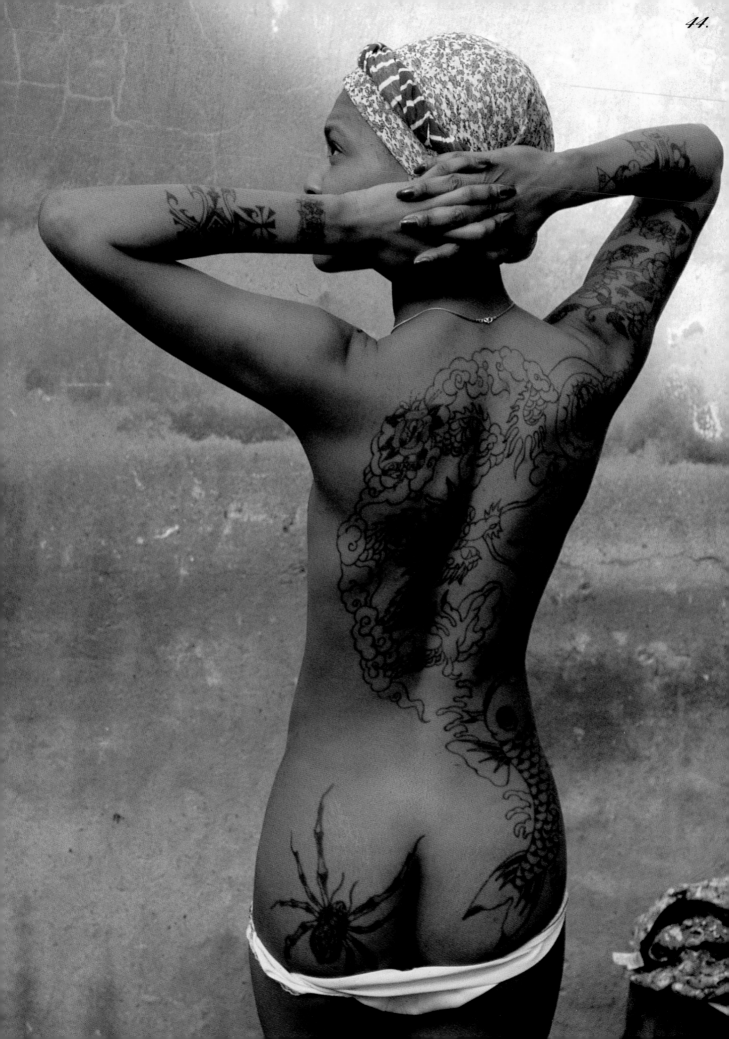

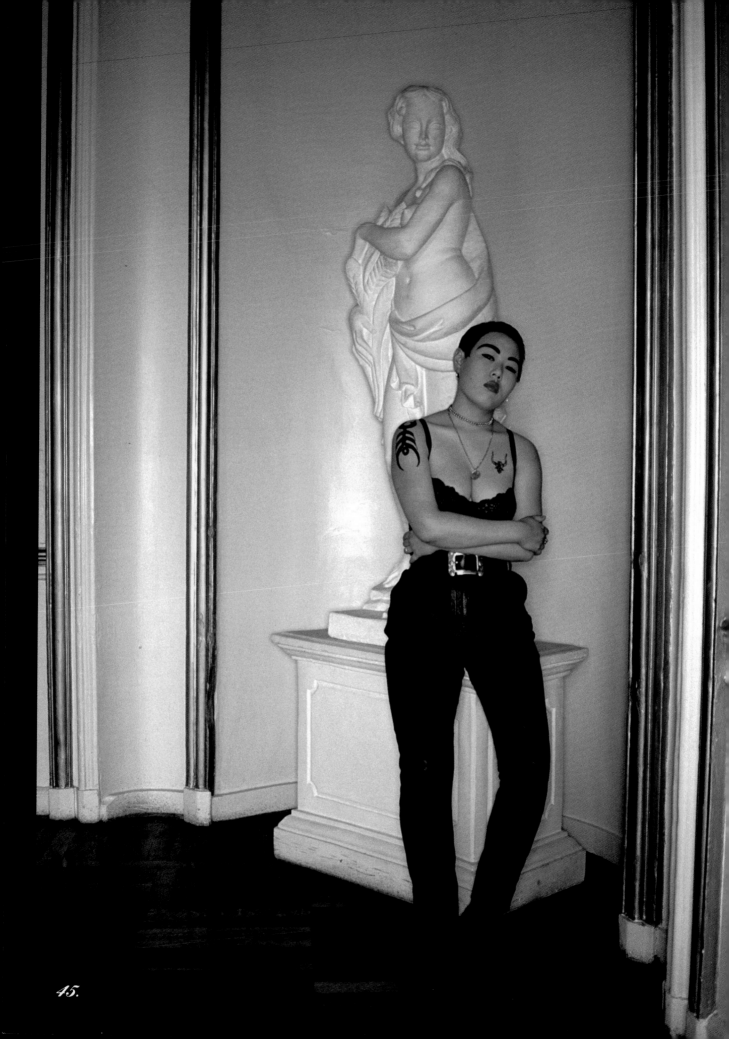

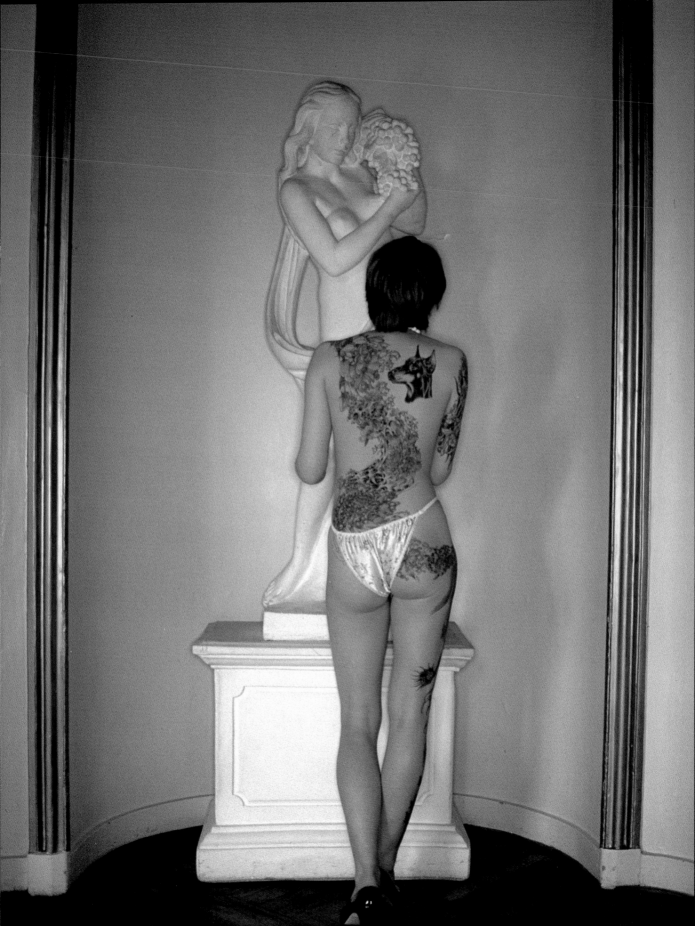

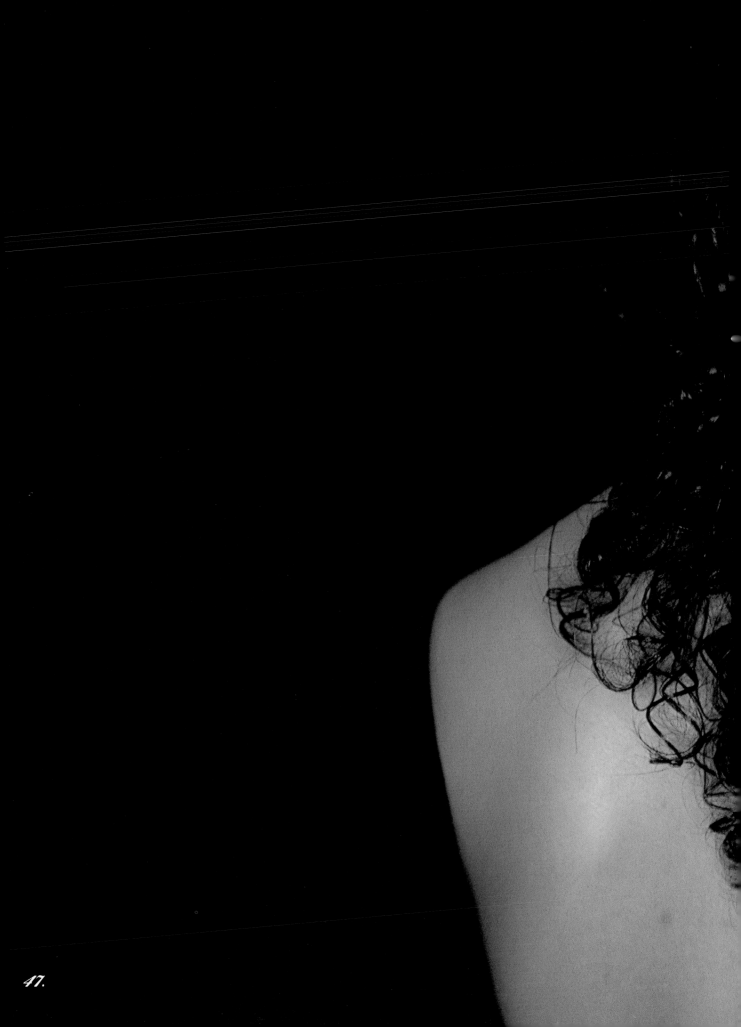

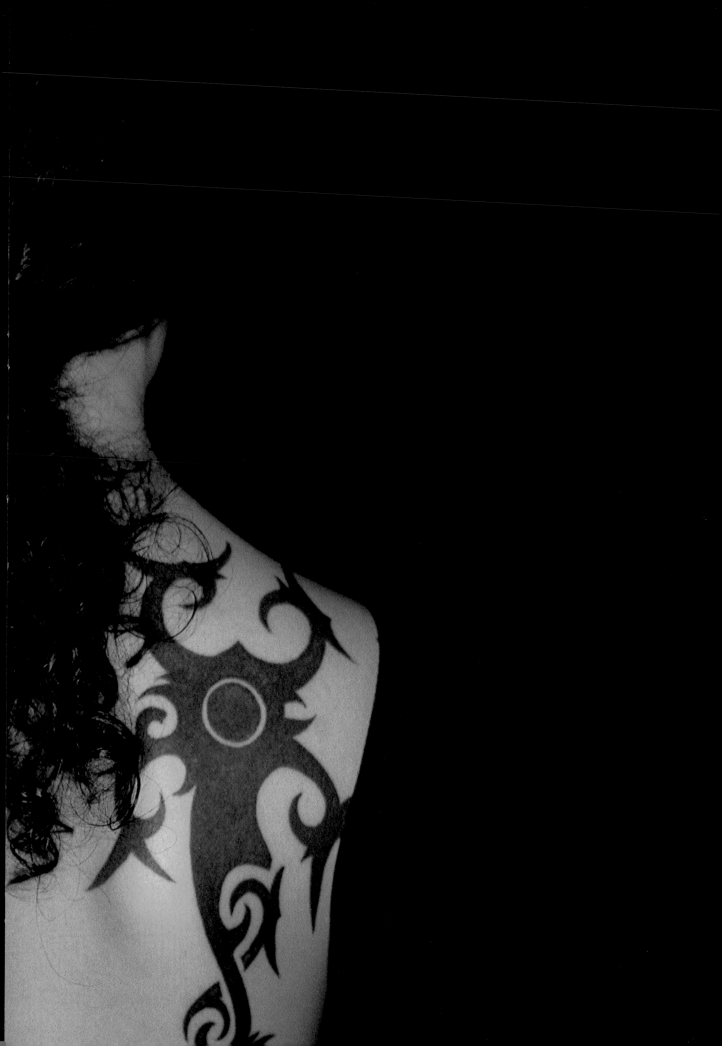

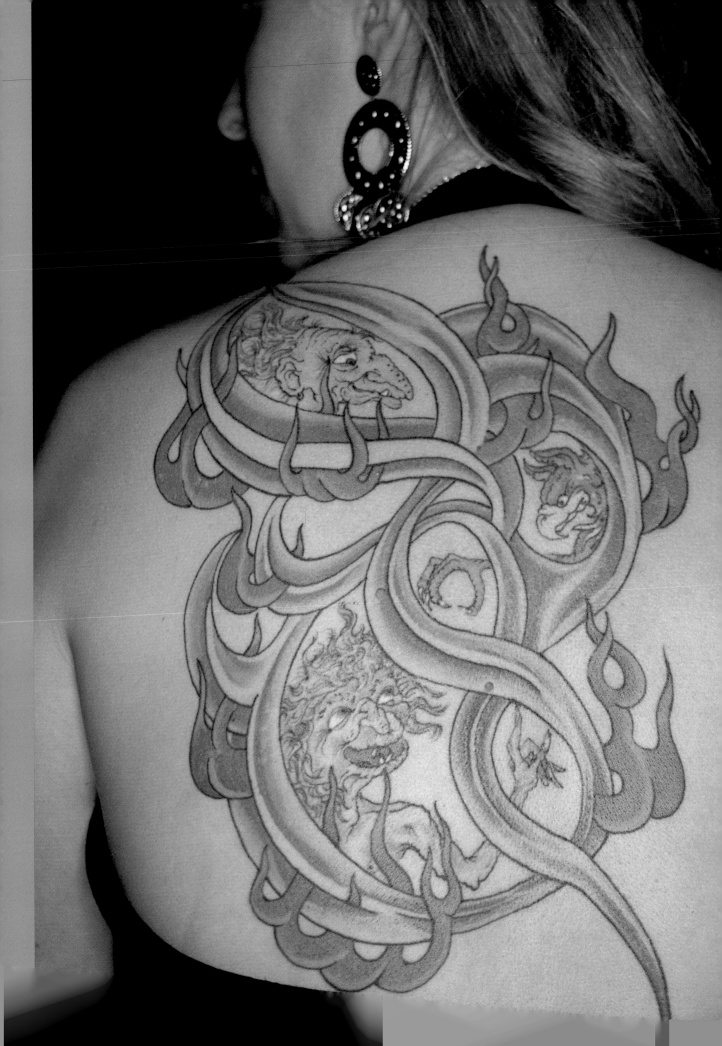

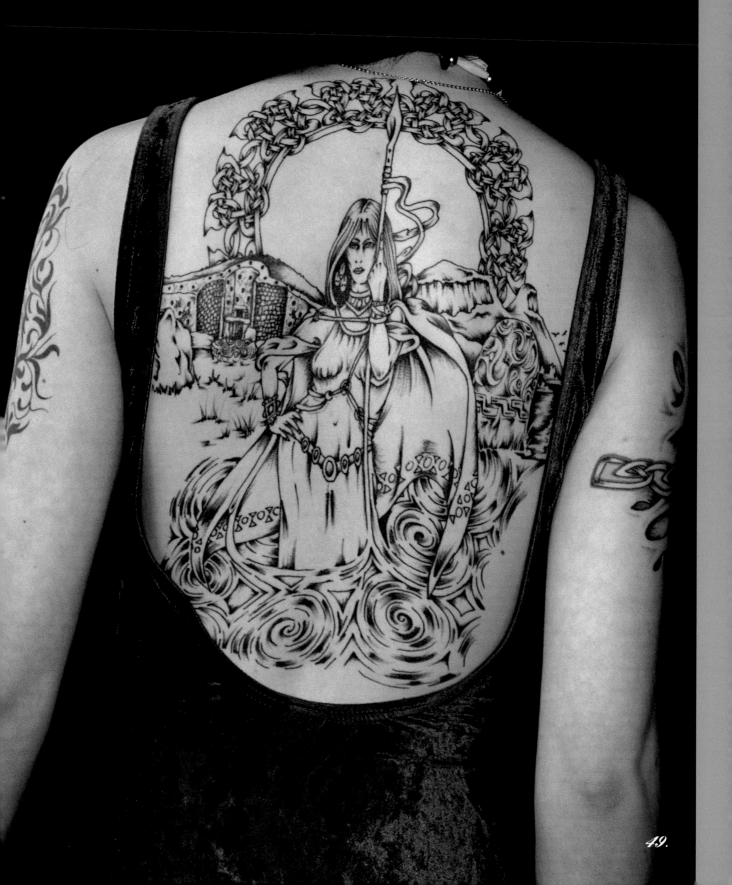

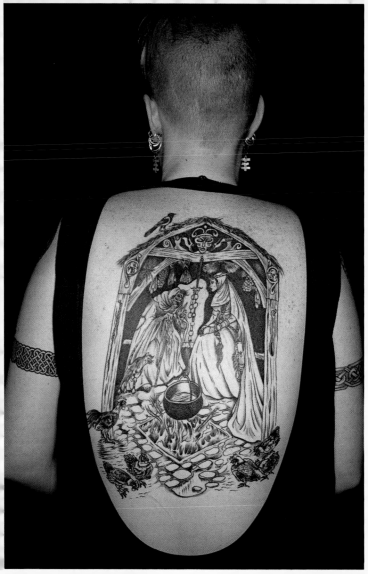

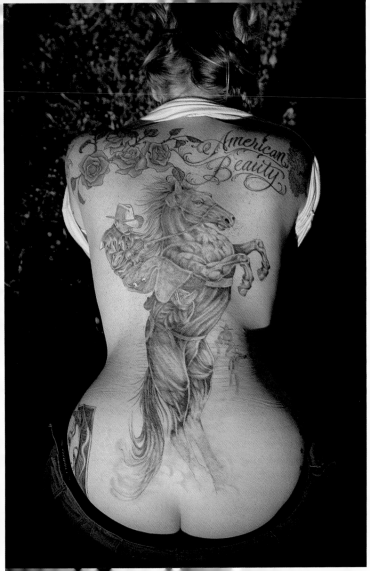

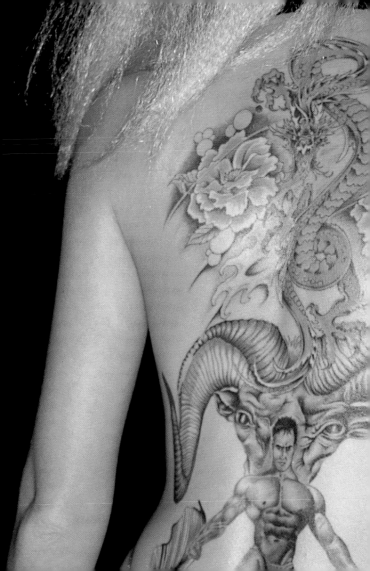

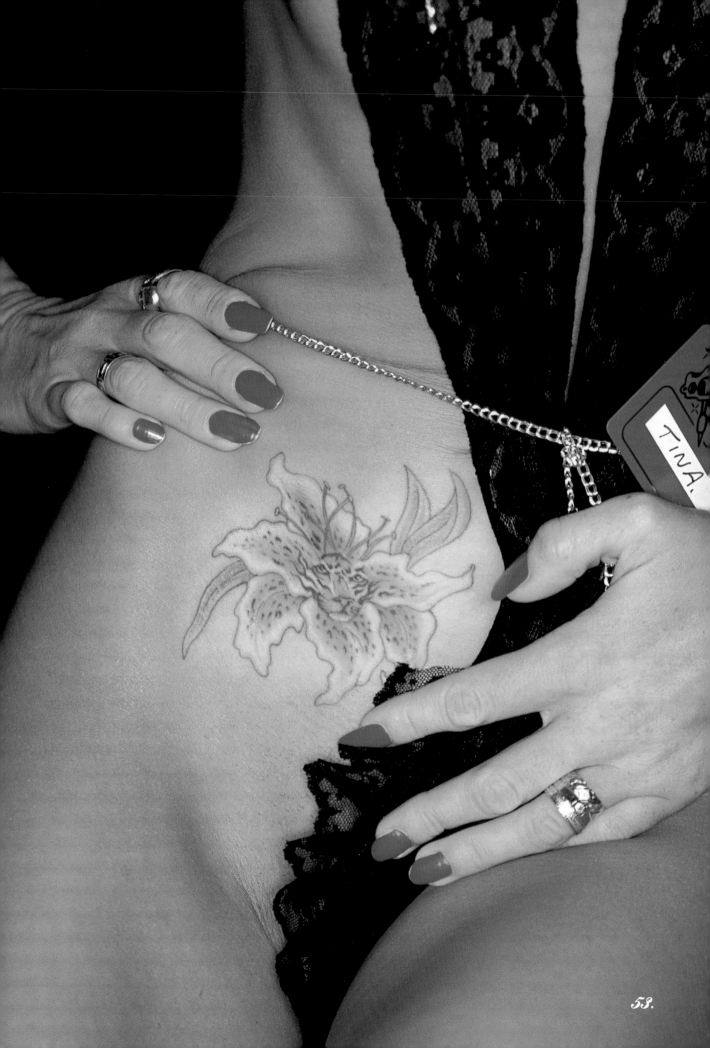

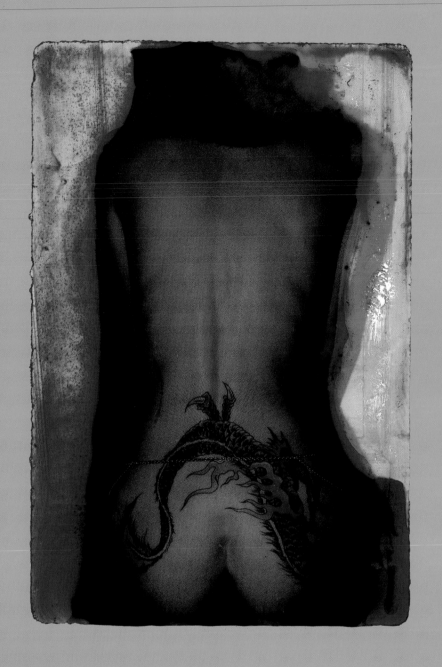

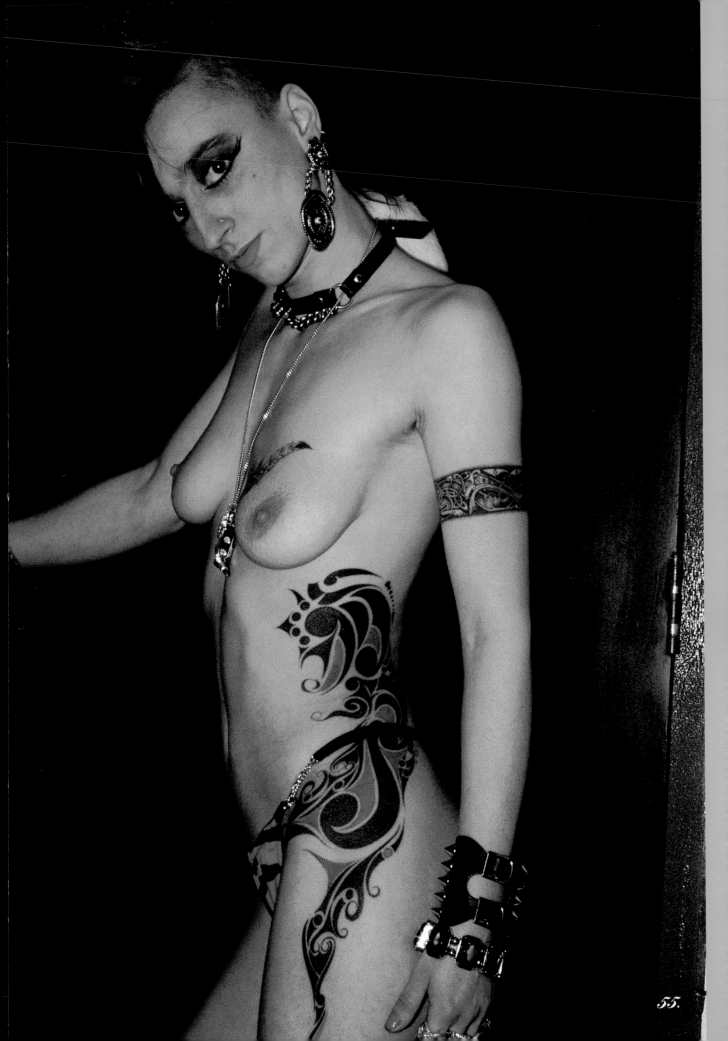

55.

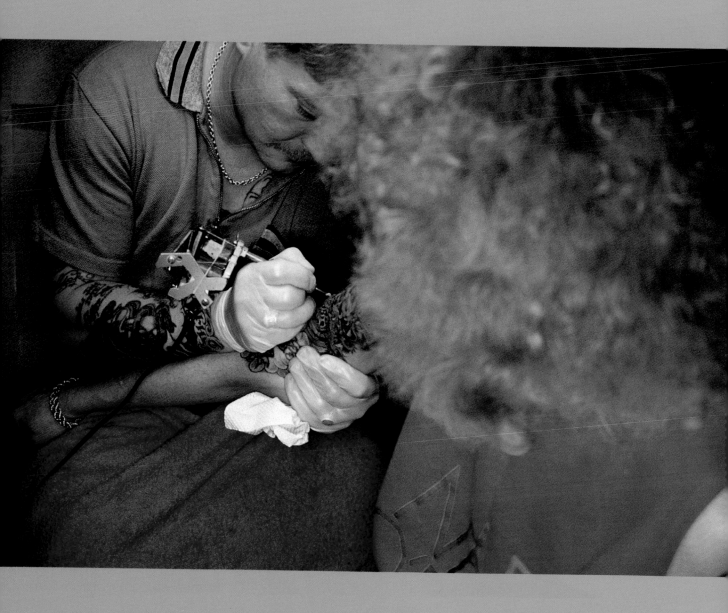

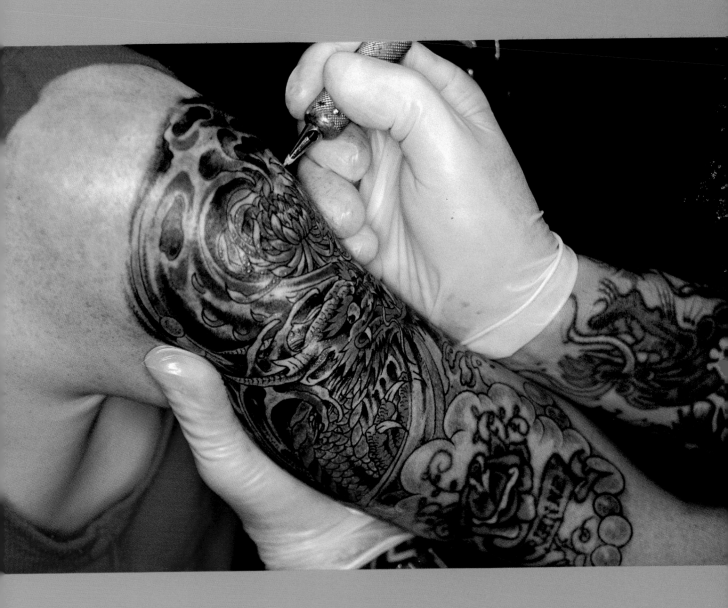

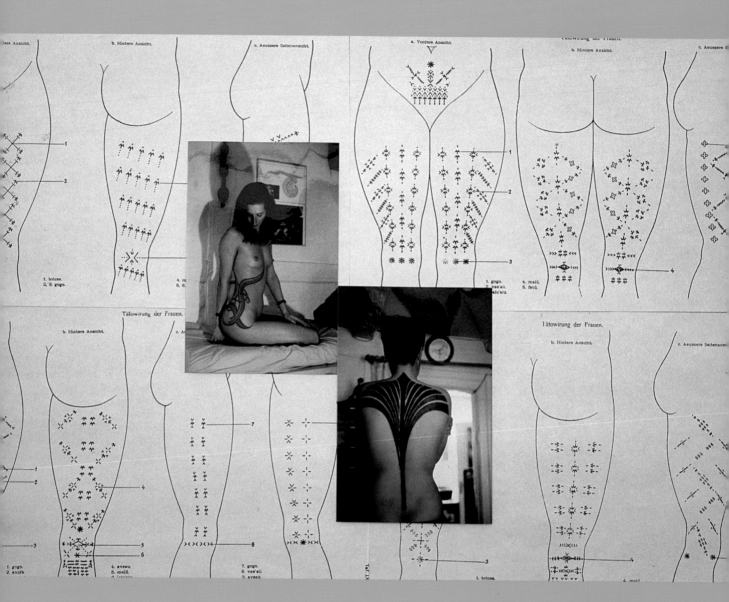

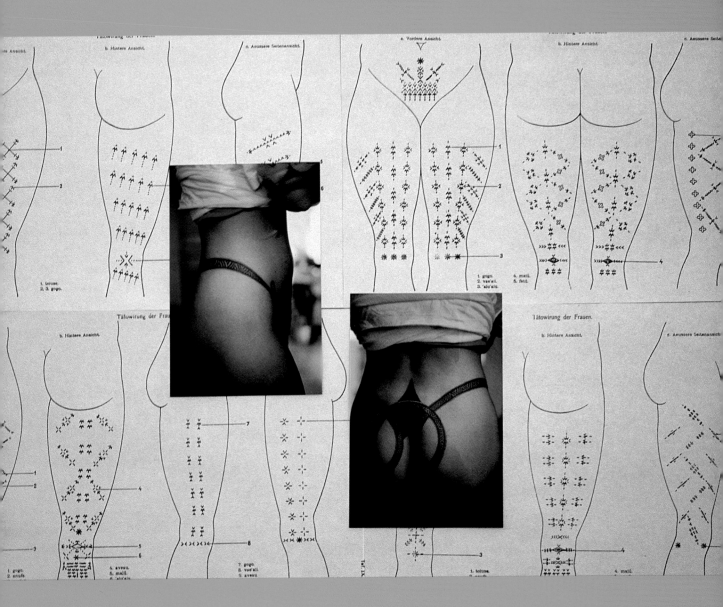

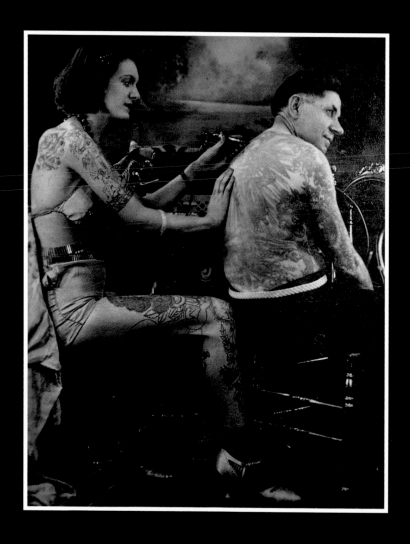

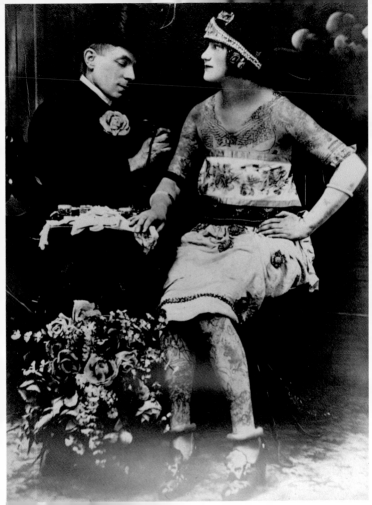

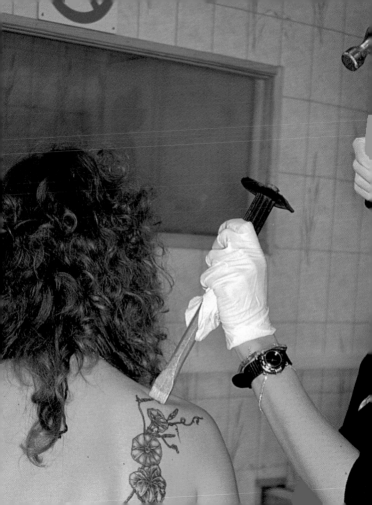

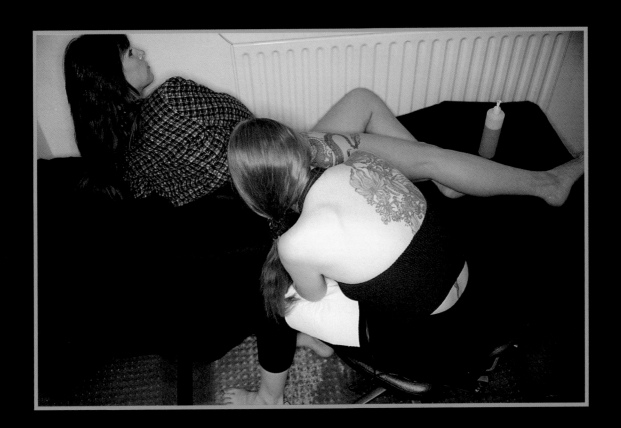

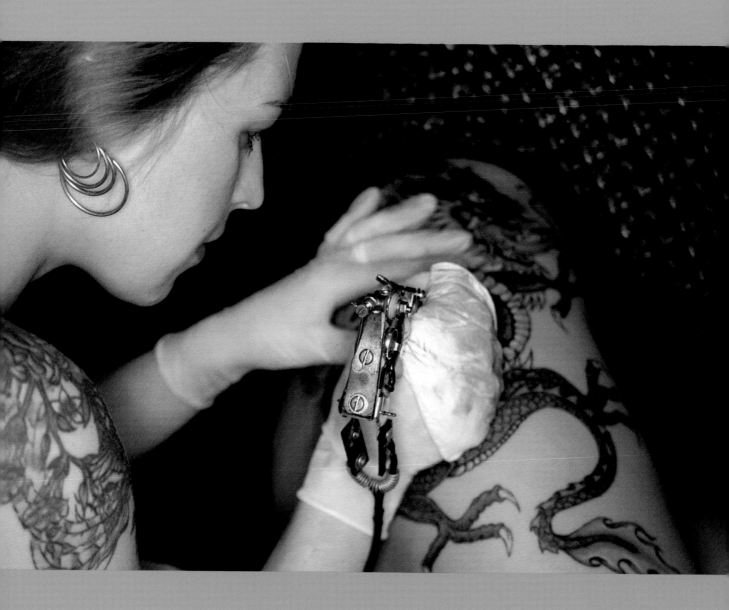

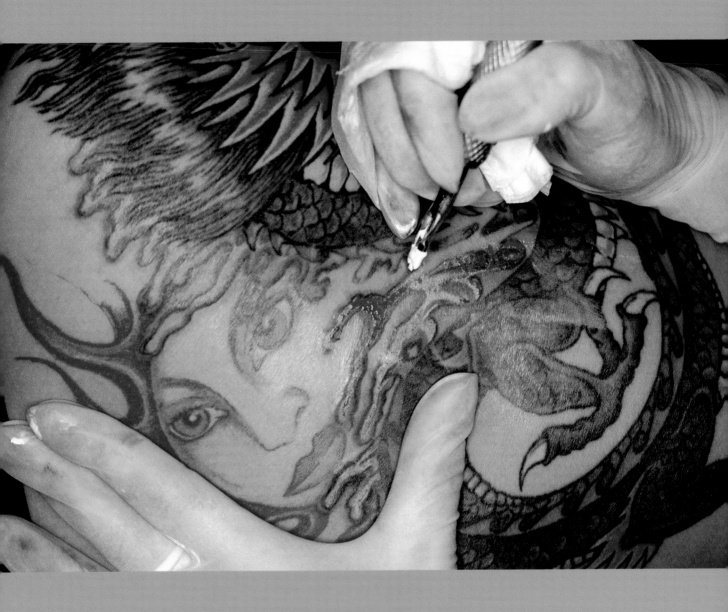

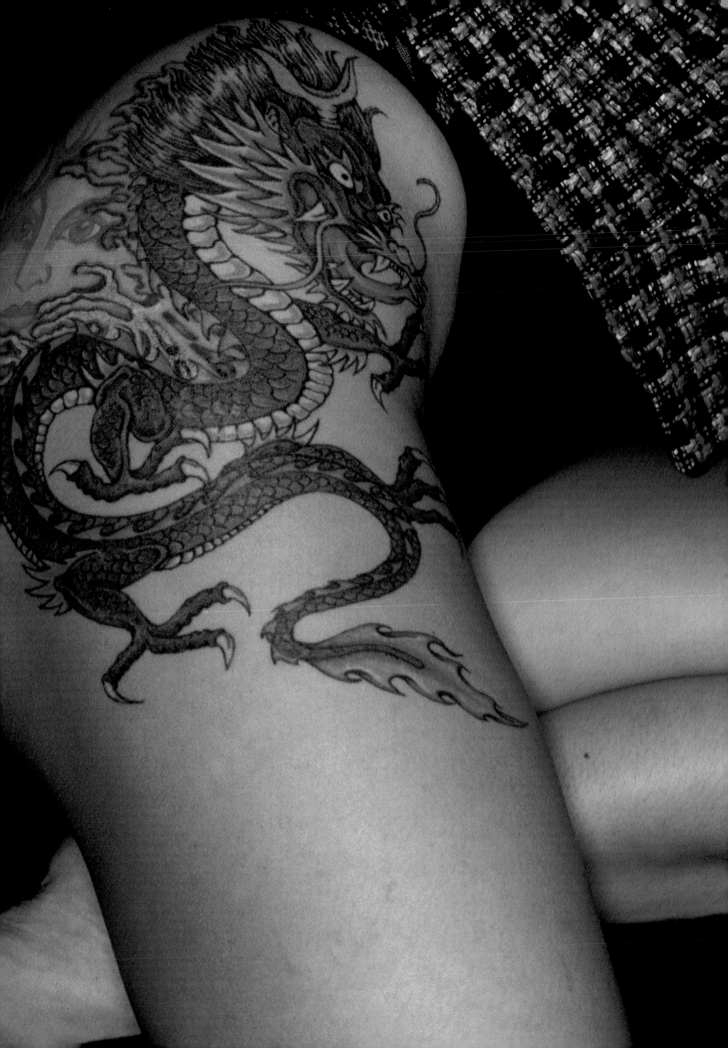

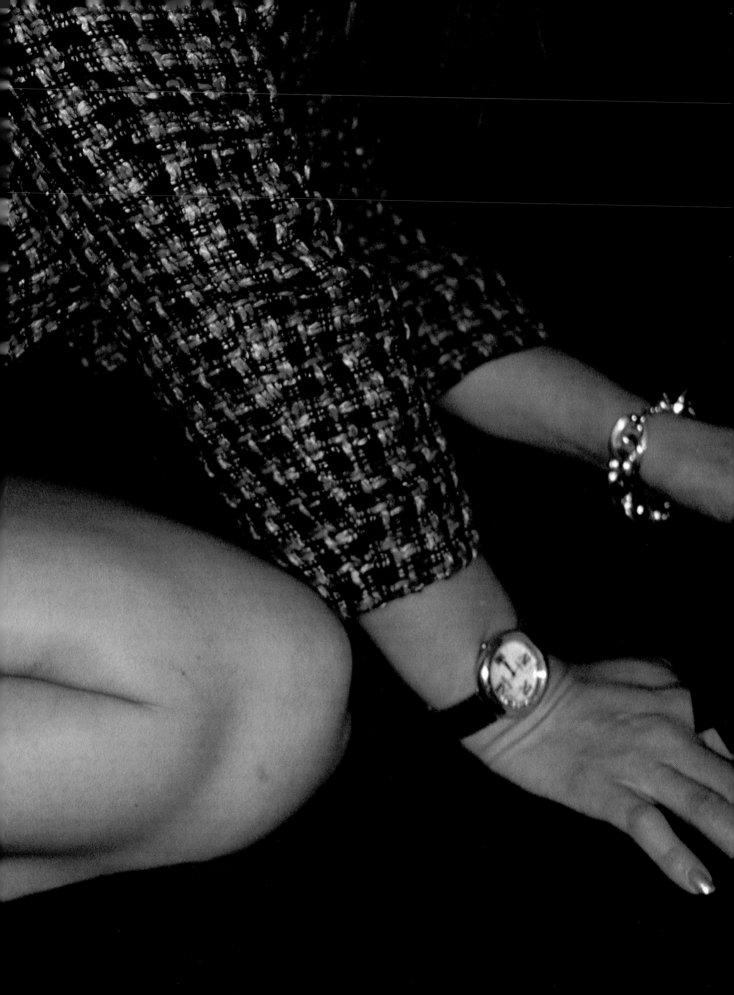

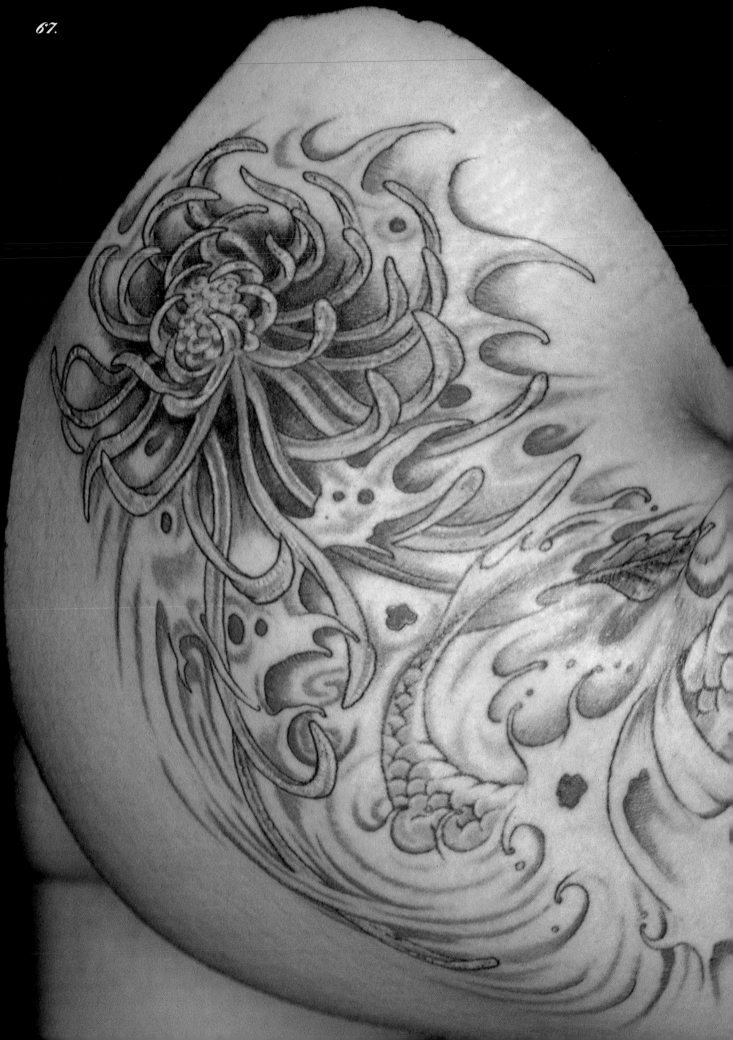

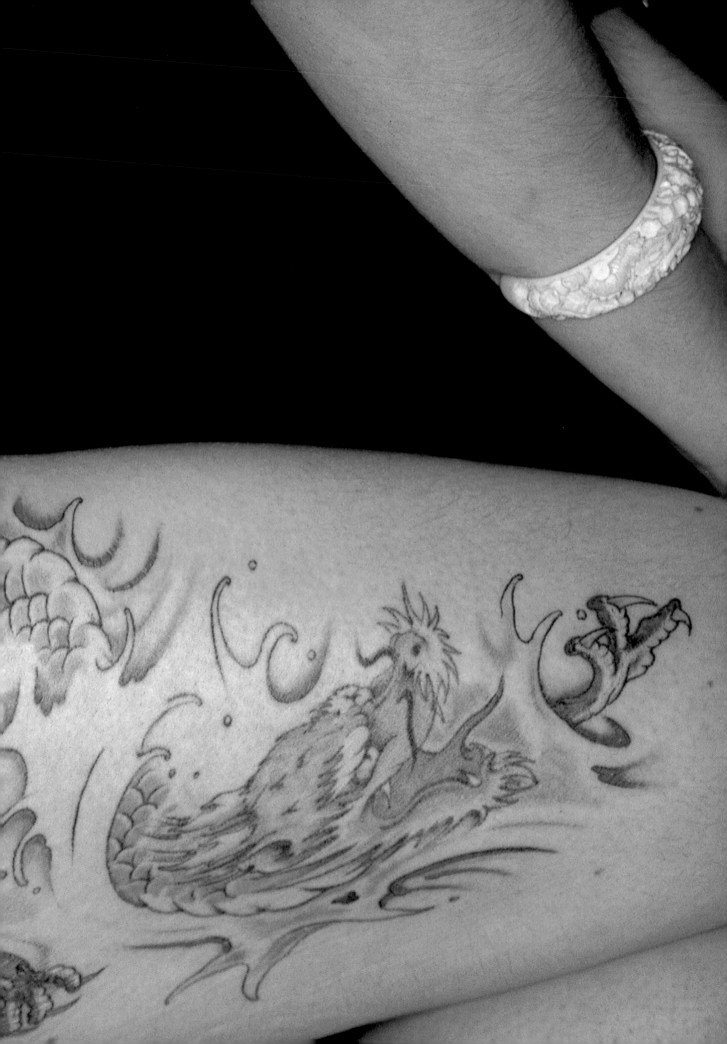

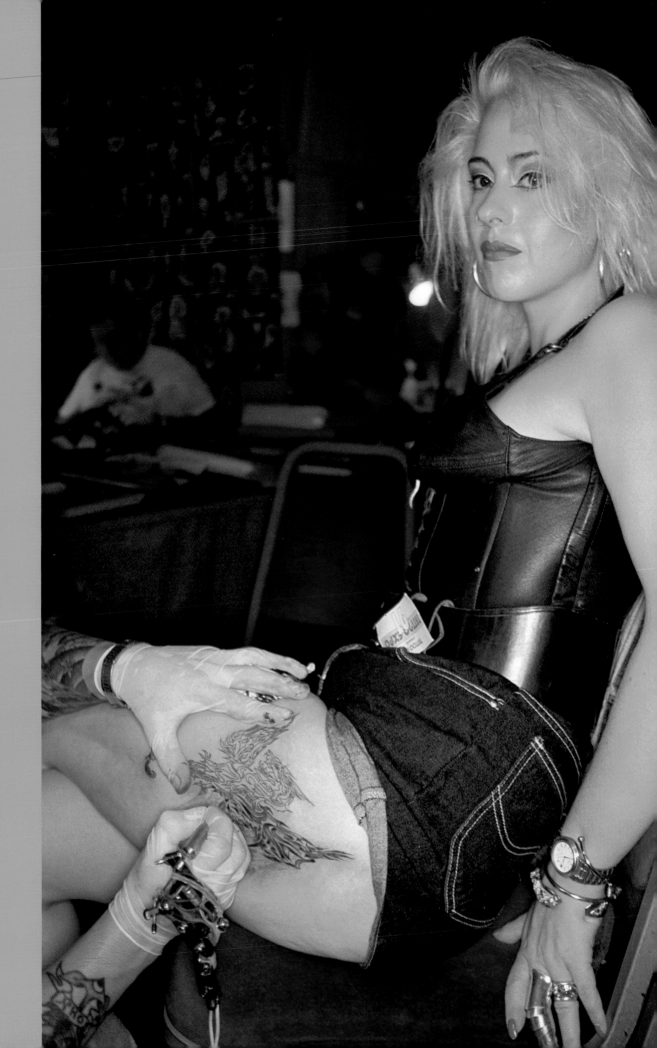

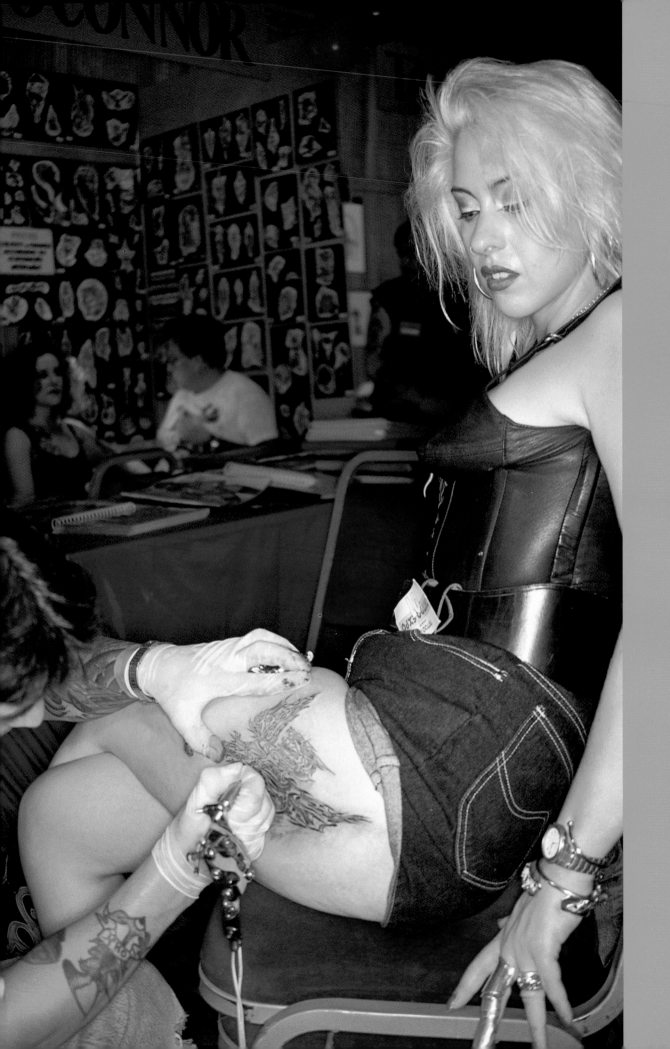

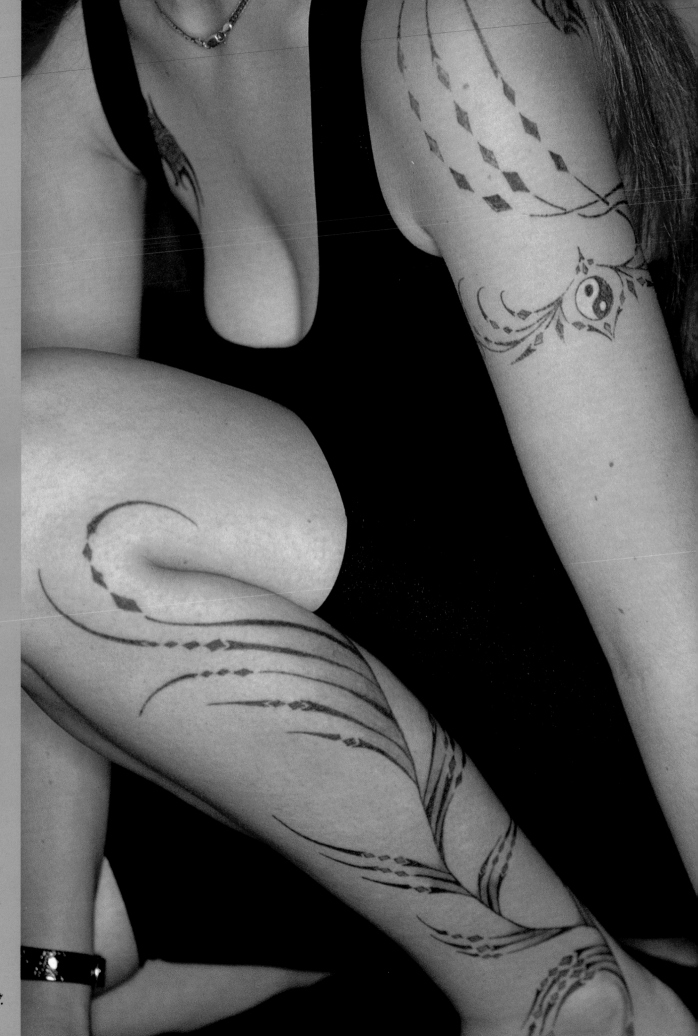

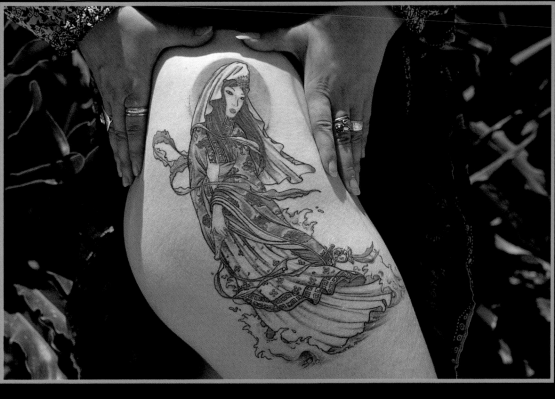

Tattooing is the mechanical introduction of pigments
under the skin, and a very well known process. The pigments
employed are carbon, cinnabar, carmine, and indigo.
 Tattooing has been practised in every country throughout
the world in various ways, from the Stone Age to the present.
In recent years, modern science has completely revolution-
ised this ancient art by the invention of the electric tattooing
instrument. The process as perfected is practically painless,
and the design is tattooed on the skin as quickly as if one
was using a fountain pen.
 Electric tattoo machines were used as early as 1891. Prof
O'Riley was the first to use the electric tattoo machine in the
United States. The electric tattoo machine is taken from the
Edison magnet vibrator movement, and will make from 1 to
3000 punctures per minute in the skin. A competent tattooist
will not be suprised at any unusual thing he may be called on
to produce, for the demands are as varied as the people who
patronise the work. The old-fashioned girl who used to show
the pictures in the red plush photo-album, now has a
daughter who lets you take a peek at the butterfly tattooed
on her leg.

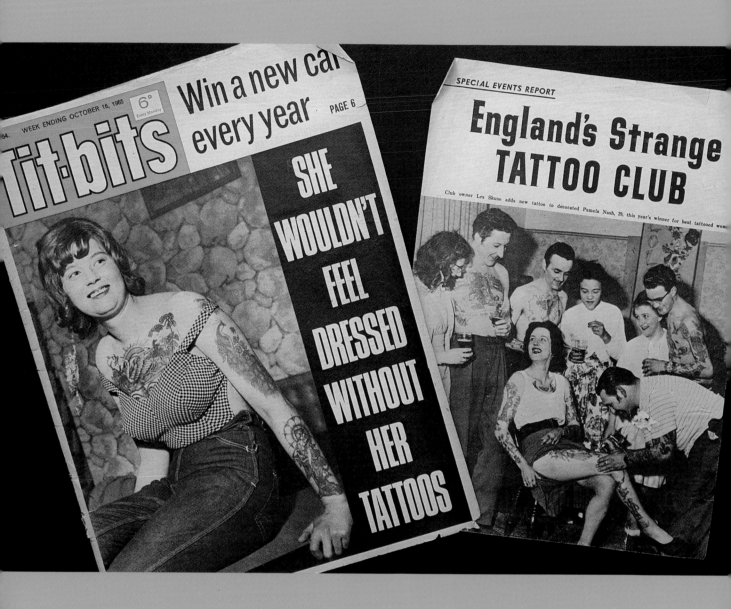

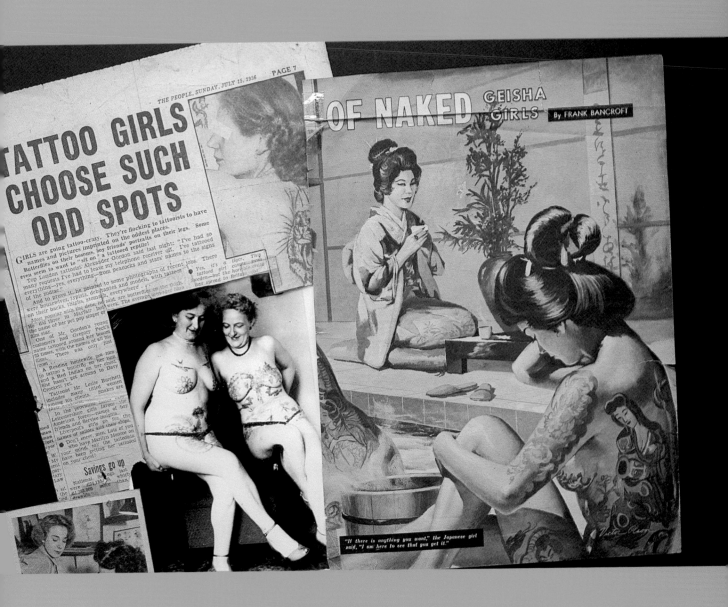

TATTOO GIRLS CHOOSE SUCH ODD SPOTS

GIRLS are going tattoo-crazy. They're flocking to tattooists to have names and pictures imprinted on the oddest places. Some Butterflies on their bosoms, boy friends' portraits on their legs.

Top London tattoist Alexander Gordon said last night: "I've tattooed even seem to want to "sit on " a tattoed reptile!

many requests I've had to leave my telephone receiver off. I've tattooed everything—yes, everything—from peacocks and stars' names to the signs of the zodiac.

And to prove it, he pointed to some photographs of recent jobs. There were housewives, typists, debutantes and models, with tattoes on their backs, thighs, stomach, everywhere • Yes, it's a tiger. The Most popular with the debs, he said, are butterflies on the thigh. tattoed girl comes from He did that in Mayfair last week. The average woman likes Sweden—but the horrible craze the name of her pet pop singer or has spread to Britain.

One Mr. Gordon's young customers had a Gregory Peck's name tattooed around her bosom six times, with the names of all his films. There was only just room.

Reading housewife got him to tattoo a butterfly on her turn and a Red Indian on her chest. She hasn't got around to Davy Crockett yet.

Tattooist Mr. Leslie Burchett includes many titled women among his clients.

In the provinces Leicestershire girls favour American forces—names of boy friends and Service insignia. Liverpool's girls go for the names of sailors and their ships.

• Don't sneer, men. Lots of you your mind. May the tattooist who have been getting her tattooks on your chest!

Savings go up

W
My
sent per-
saw
National
were £91,158.2
the £1,538,869
tied. £

OF NAKED GEISHA GIRLS   By FRANK BANCROFT

"If there is anything you want," the Japanese girl said, "I am here to see that you get it."

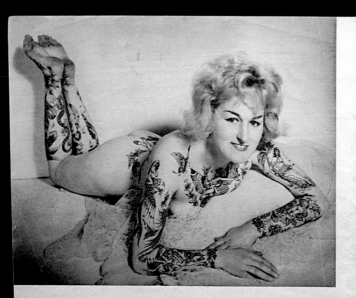

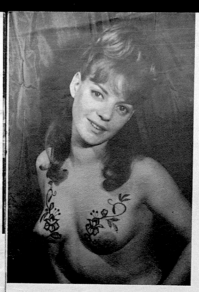

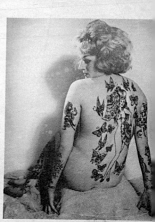

UNCOVERING variety of artistic designs (left, above), tattooed ladies bare handiwork.

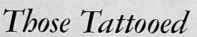

Those Tattooed   Ladies...

By Cindy Ray
As told to Arch Ayres

Proving that tattooing is not lost art, Australia's painted doll discloses secrets of exotic needlework while promoting its world-wide acceptance.

LOUNGING on delicate lace, Cindy Ray shows extent of artwork on her body (top). LEFT: Donning wig, she proves tattoos are complement to any shade of hair and because of multi-shaped designs can feature variety of shadings.

26   • MODERN MAN •

TO MOST PEOPLE, a few tattoos on a man represents a rugged sort of masculinity. In fact, military men consider them as lifetime "badges" of their profession, long after a hitch is served, when the uniform becomes many sizes too small.

But, unfortunately, society raises a startled eyebrow when a tattooed lady appears on the scene. She's considered "freakish" and is snubbed like the proverbial plague. Since I've become known as the "tattooed lady," however, I have found this attitude to be generally disappearing—particularly in my native Australia, where more and more women are appearing in public with multi-colored tattoos on their arms and legs and, as these photos indicate, other areas of the anatomy, as well.

When I'm asked, "What made you decide to get tattooed all over?" I generally answer that it was done for three reasons: First, I got tattooed for fun; second, I

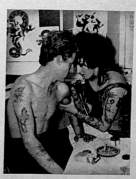

GIVING pointers at close quarters (above) is fun for tattooist if client is shapely female but sensation of needle becomes almost unbearable after few sessions of intricate shading.

• MODERN MAN •   27

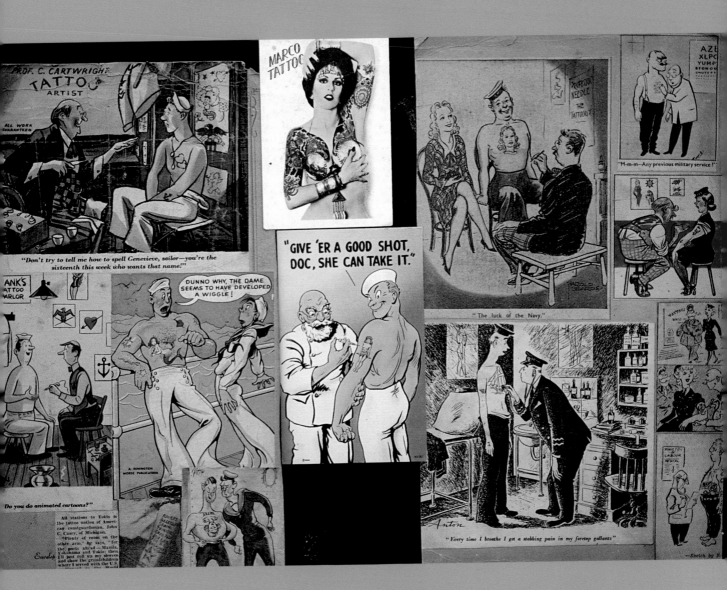

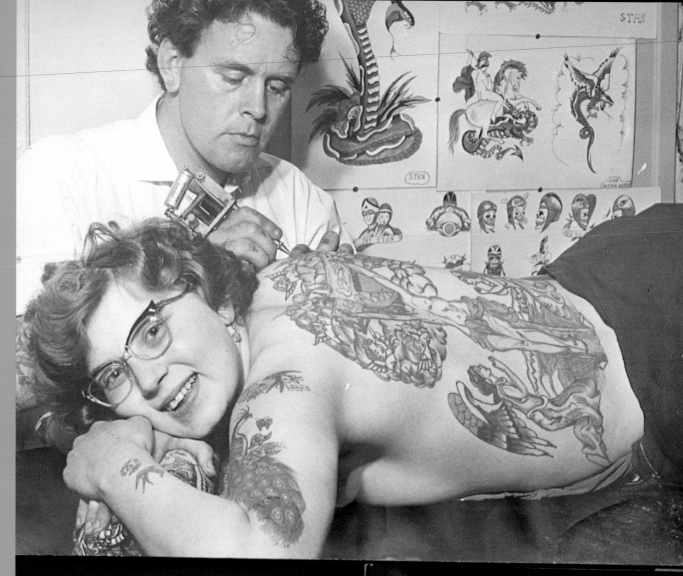

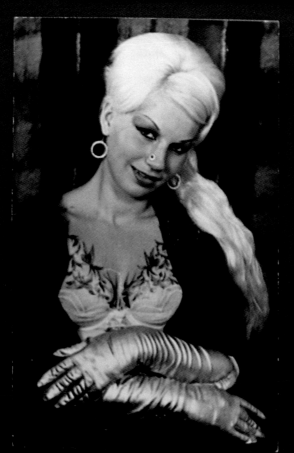

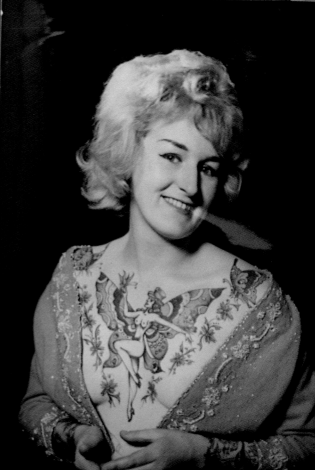

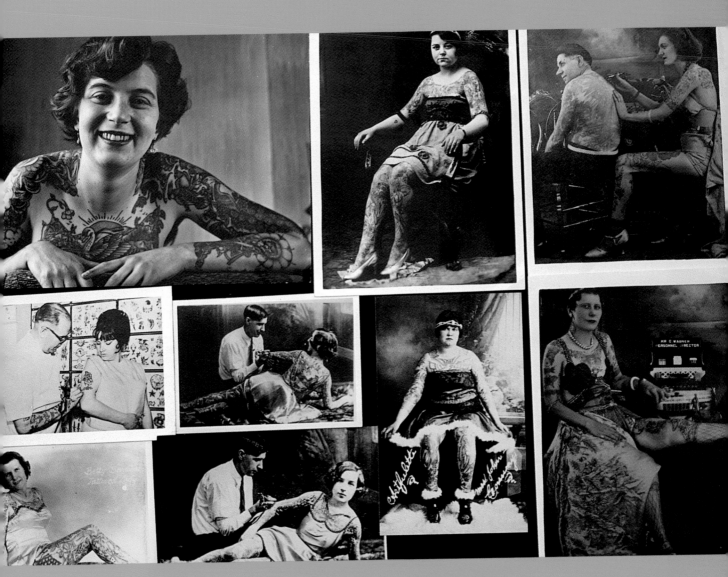

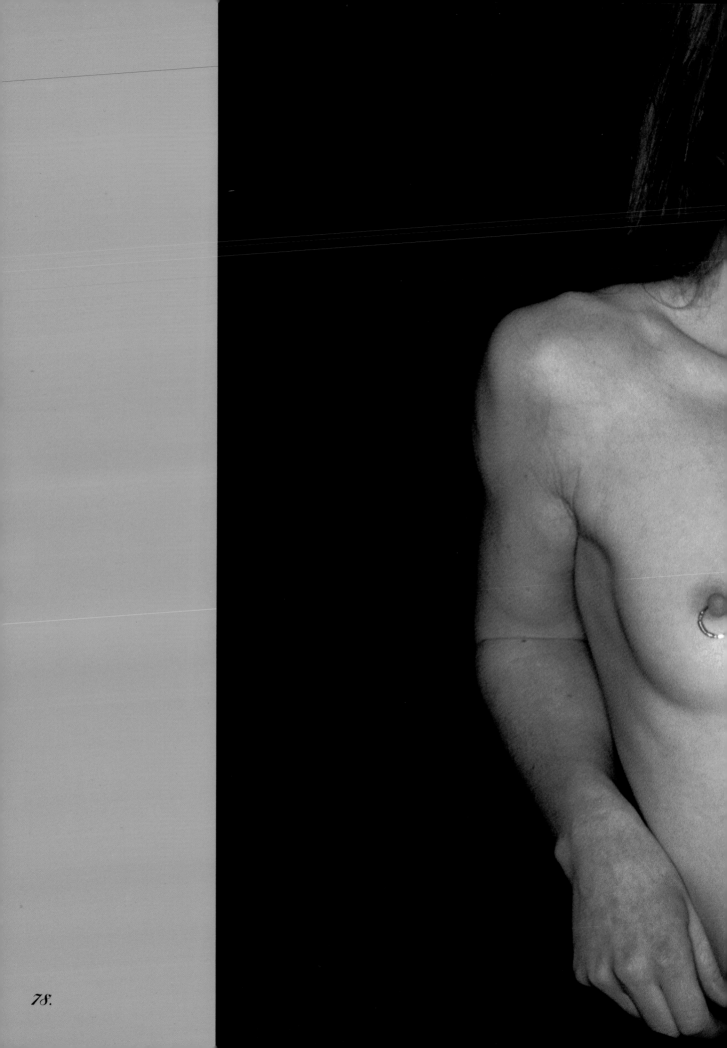

78.

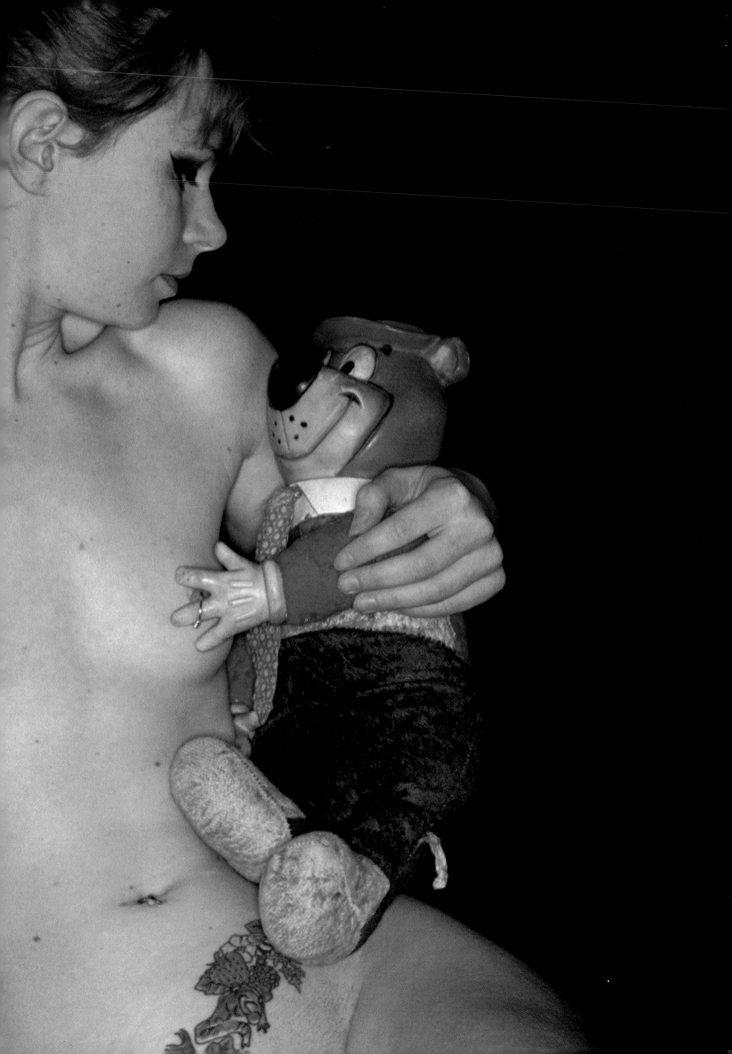

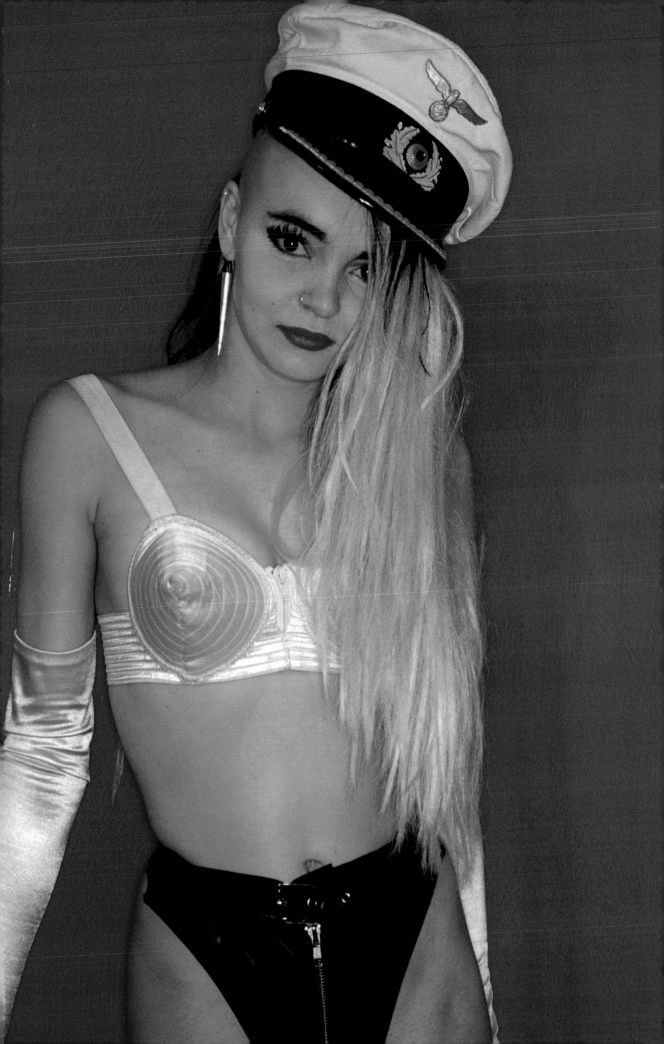

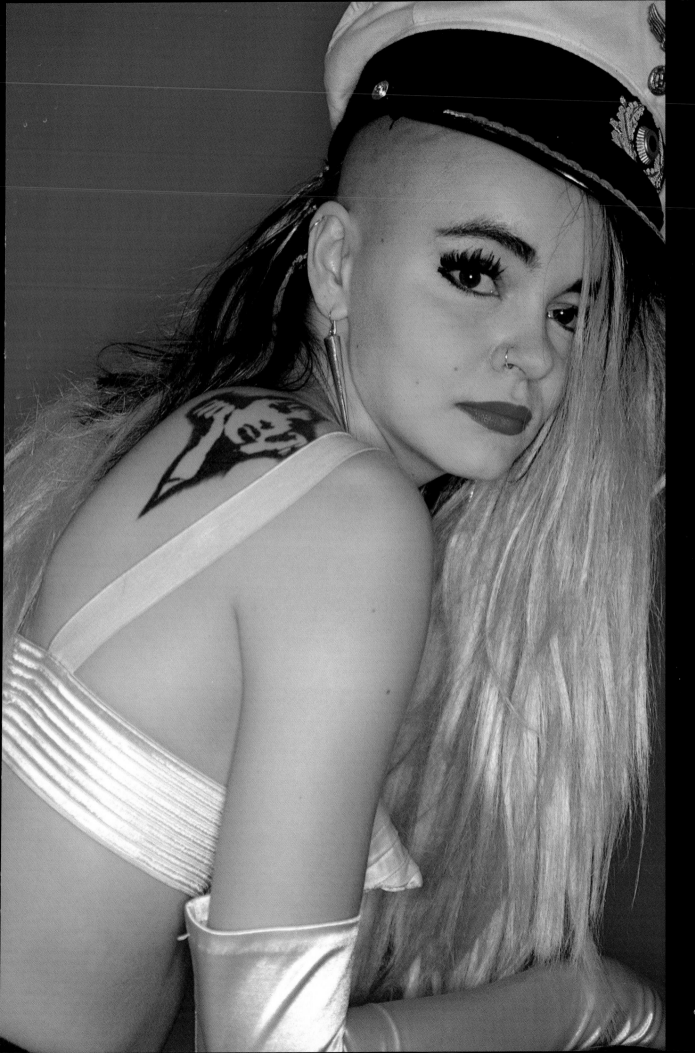

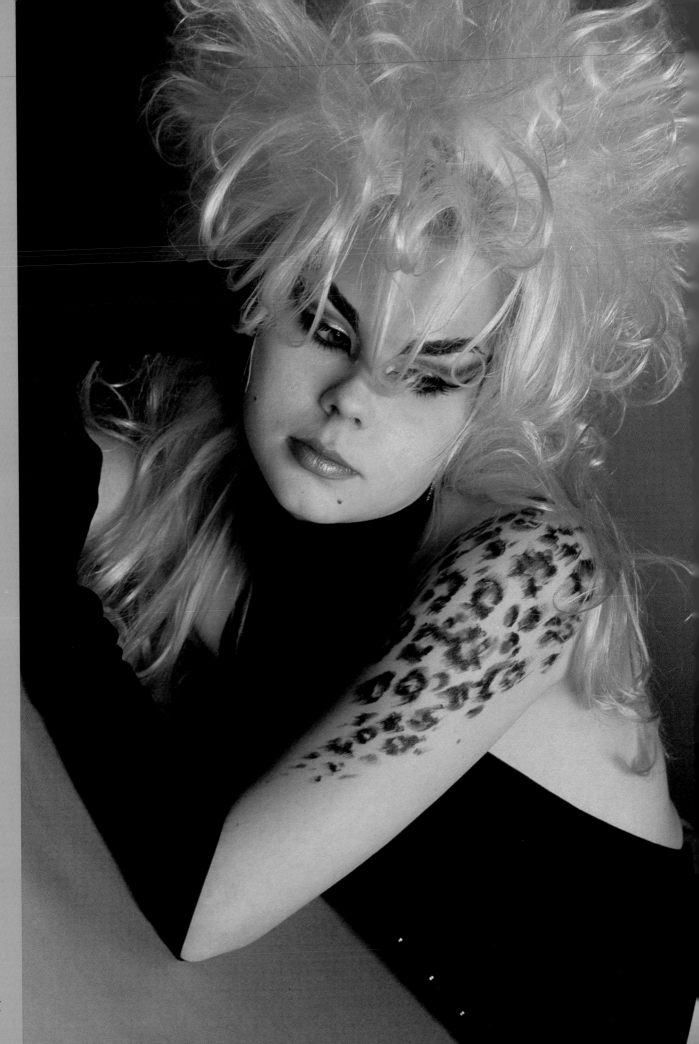

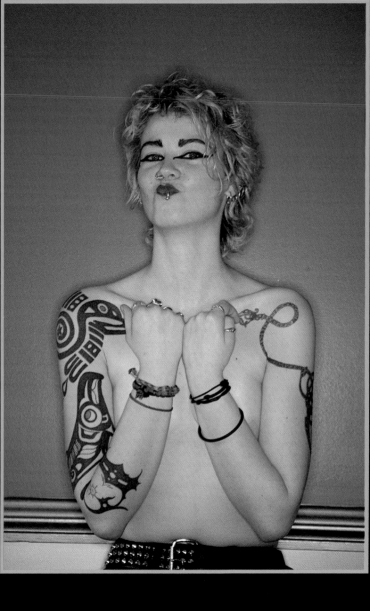

To most people, a few tattoos on a man represent a rugged sort of masculinity. In fact, military men consider them as a lifetime of 'badges' of their profession, long after the hitch is served, when their uniform becomes many sizes too small.

But unfortunately, society raises a startled eyebrow when a tattooed lady appears on the scene. She's considered 'freakish' and is snubbed like the proverbial plague. Since I've become known as the "tattooed lady", however, I have found this attitude to be generally disappearing - particularly in my native Australia, where more and more women are appearing in public with multi-coloured tattoos on their arms and legs, and, as these photographs indicate, other areas of the anatomy as well.

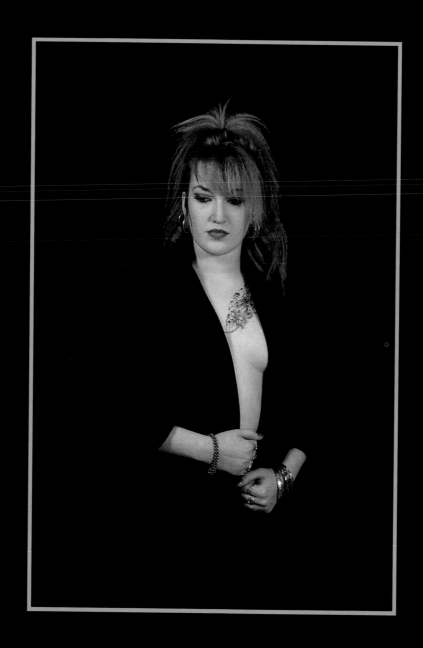

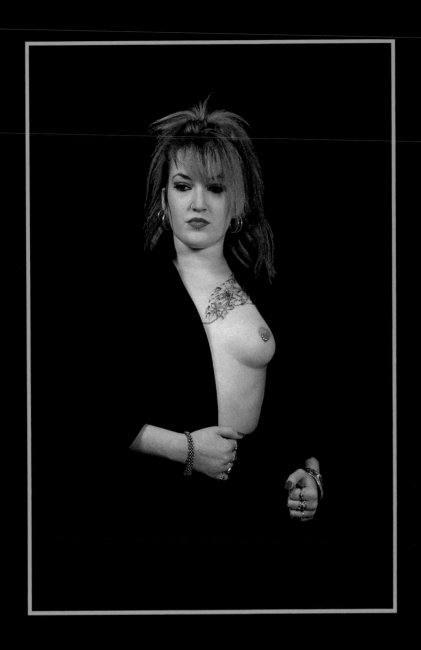

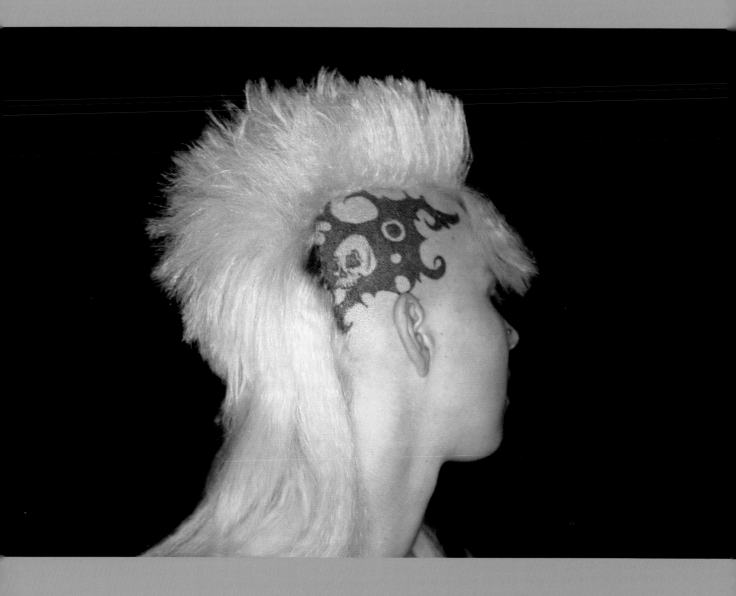

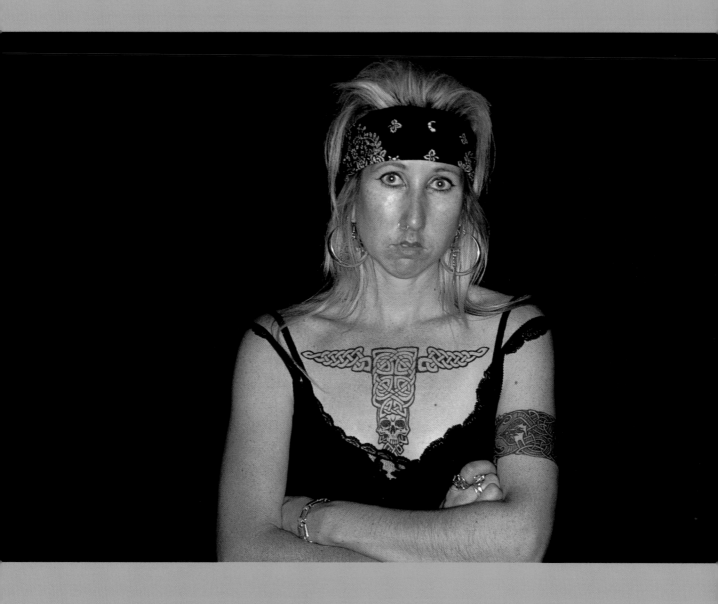

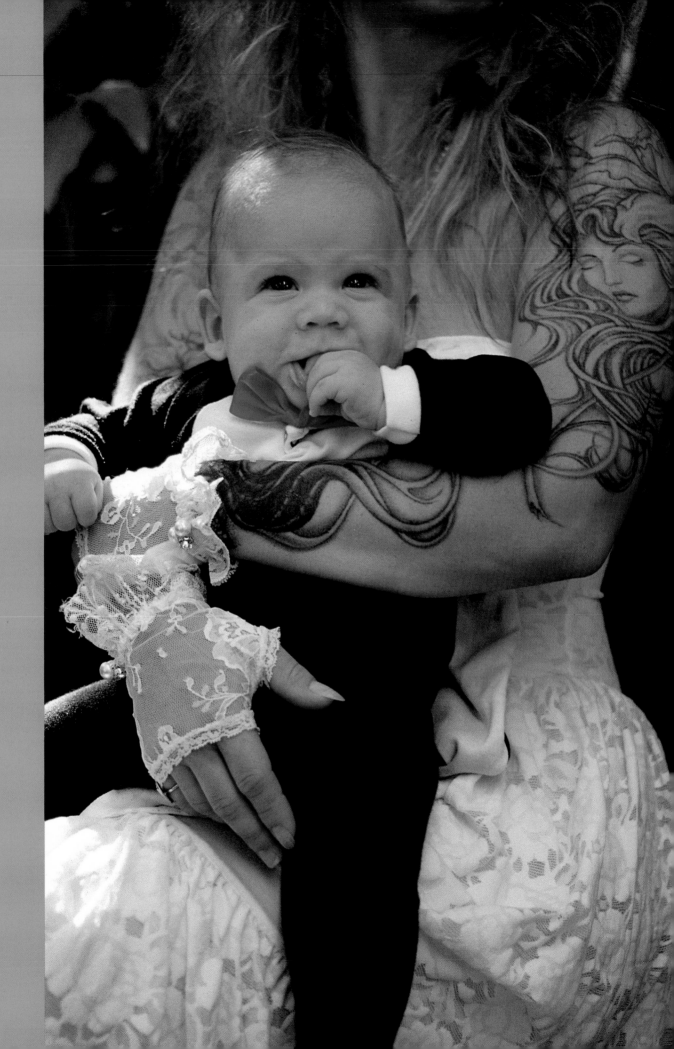

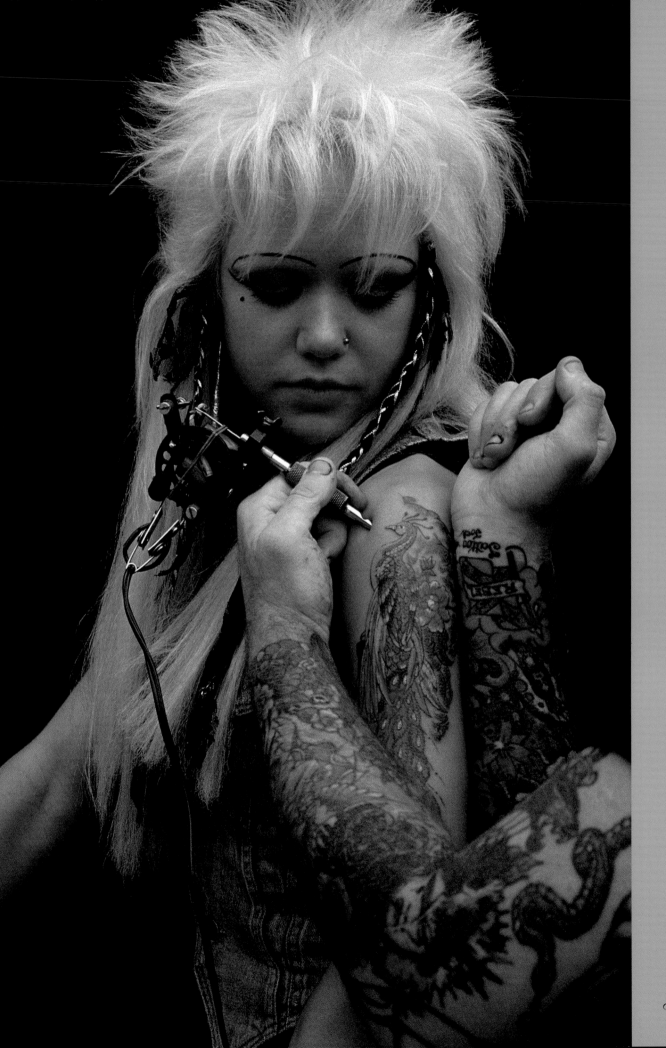

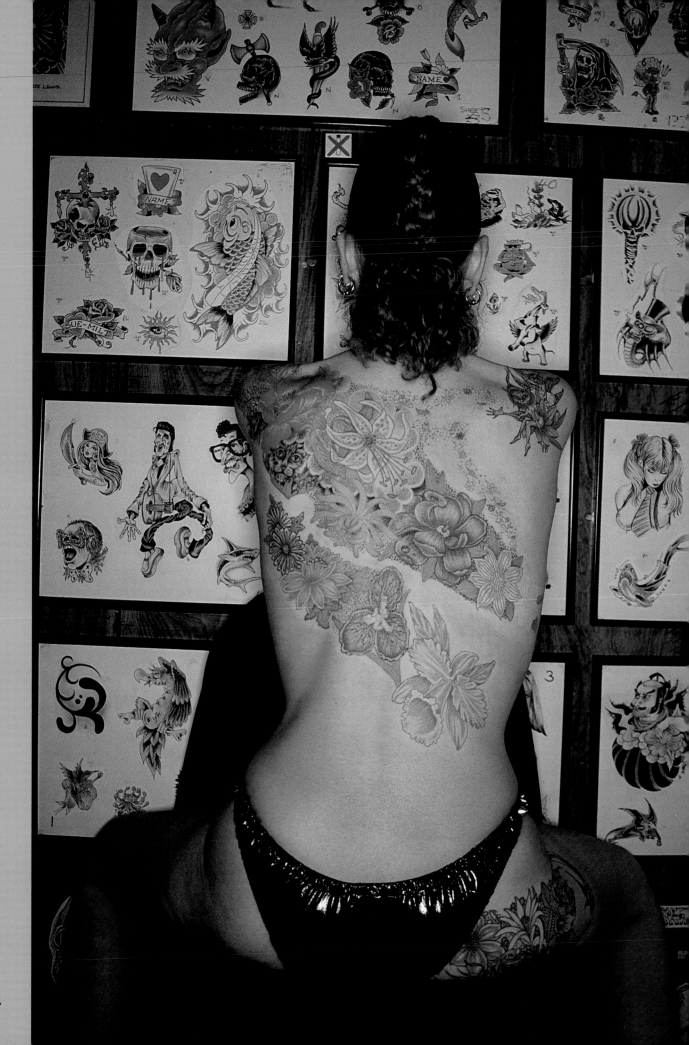

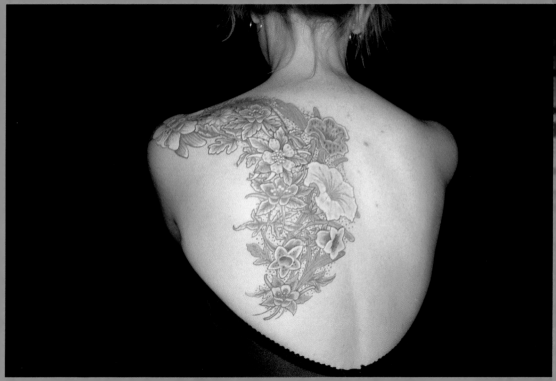

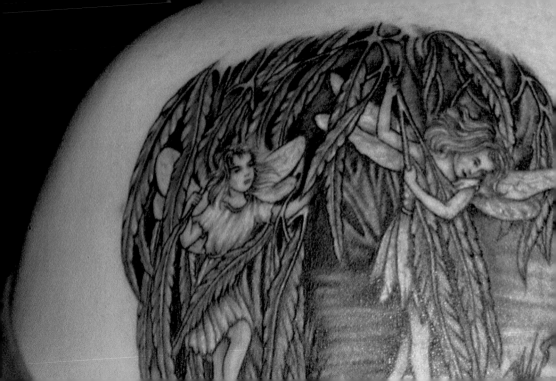

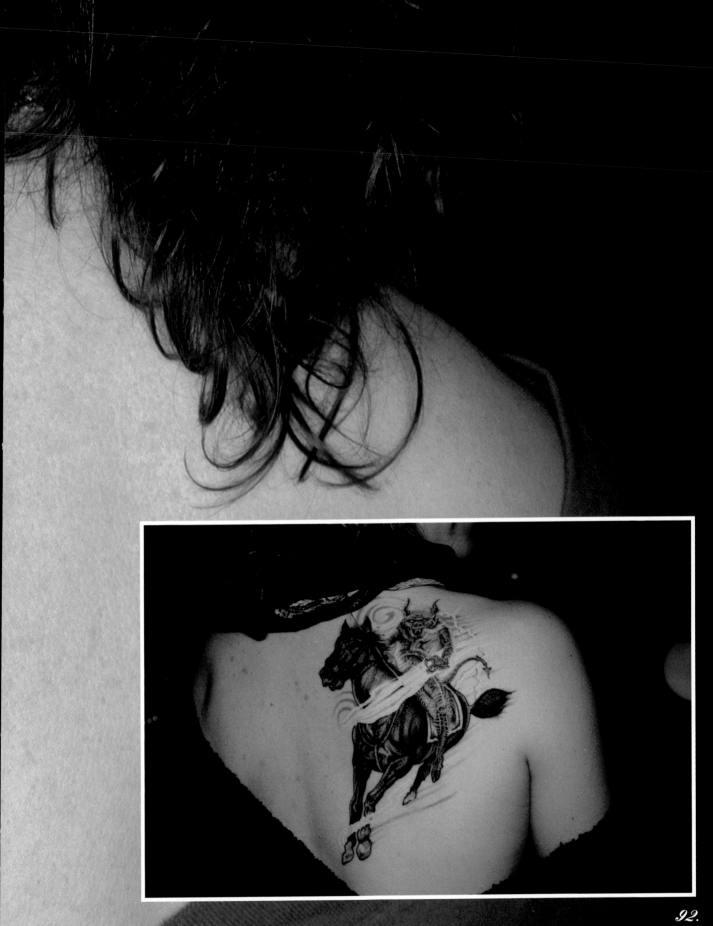

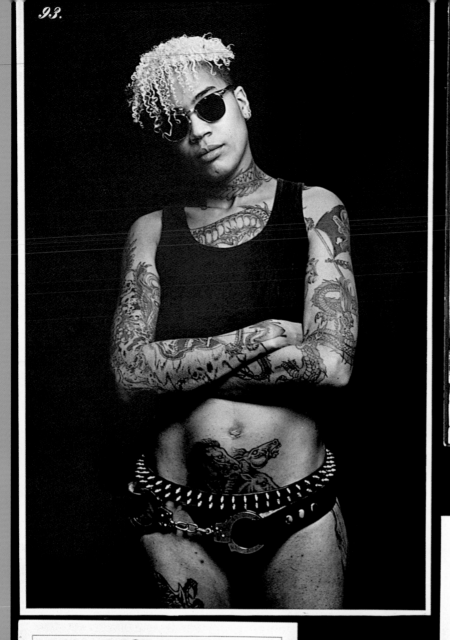

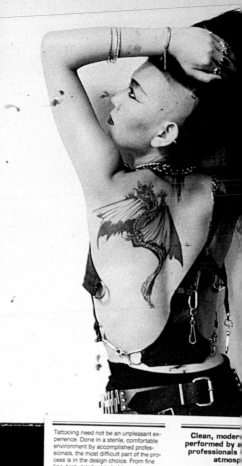

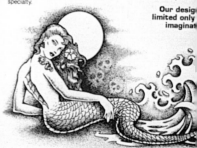

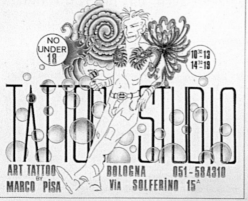

NO UNDER 18

10 DE 13 14 DE 19

ART TATTOO BY MARCO PISA BOLOGNA Via SOLFERINO 15ᴬ 051-584310

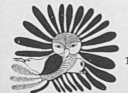

KUNSTEN PÅ KROPPEN

TATOVERING
V/ ERIK REIME
GL.MØNT 35,I
1117 KØBENHAVN K
tlf. 33 14 48 26

Åbent: Man. - Fredag 11-18.00 Samt efter aftale

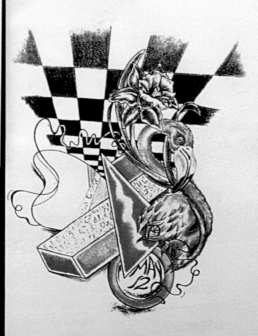

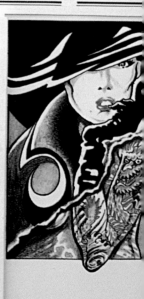

CHUCK'S CUSTOM TATTOOS

22 Goresbrook Road
Dagenham
Essex RM9 6UR
081 - 984 0013

Artwork, Crafts and Body Art
Female Tattoo Artist
Registered with Local Health Authority

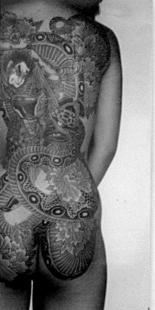

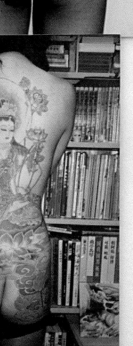

I ♥ MY TATTOO

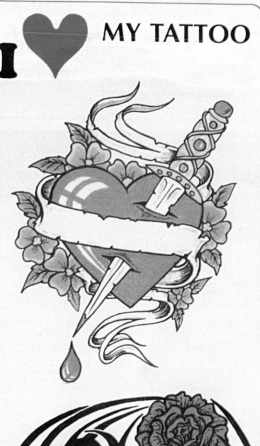

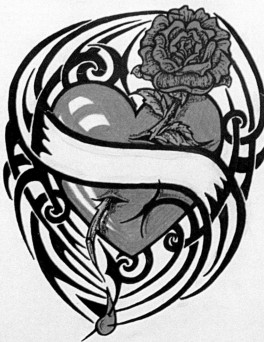

MAGIC TATTOO

ARIES STUDIO

NO PHONE

320 Kuulei KAILUA

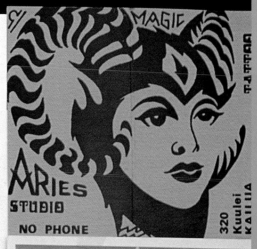

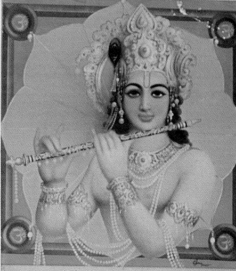

LET US TAKE HIGHER
EDEN HASHISH CENTRE
Phone : 13863

Oldest & Favourite Shop in Town Serving you the Best Nepalese Hash & Ganja
(Available Wholesale & Retail)
COME VISIT US ANY TIME FOR ALL YOUR HASHISH NEEDS
EDEN HASHISH CENTRE
OLD 5/1, Bashantpur, KATHMANDU
NEW 5/259, Ombahal, NEPAL
Prop. D. D. SHARMA

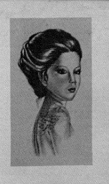

Madam Lazonga's
Dermagraphics
5485 Mission Street
San Francisco, CA 94112
(415) 333-9203

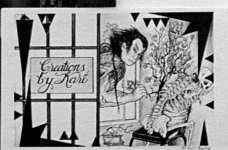

Creations by Kari

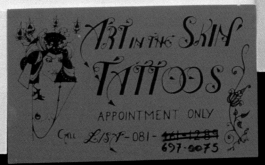

ART IN THE SKIN
TATTOOS
APPOINTMENT ONLY
CALL LISA-081-4411289
697-0075

94.

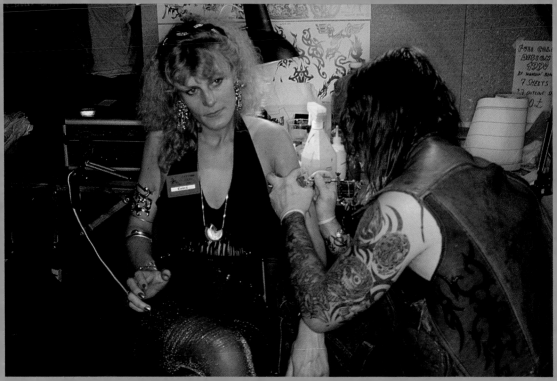

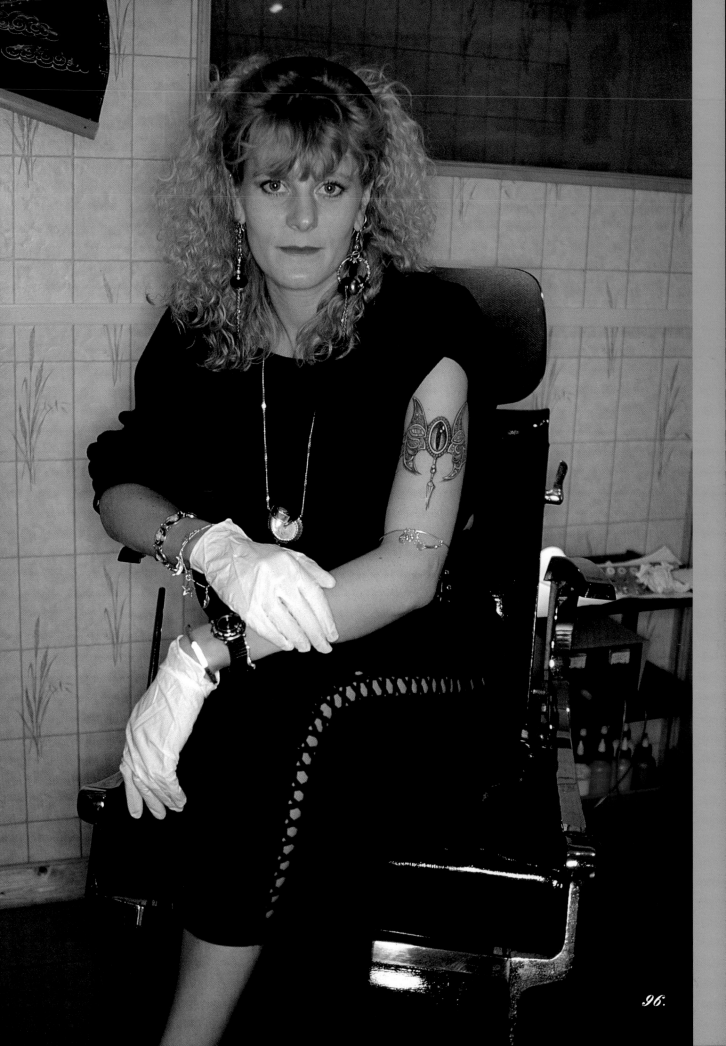

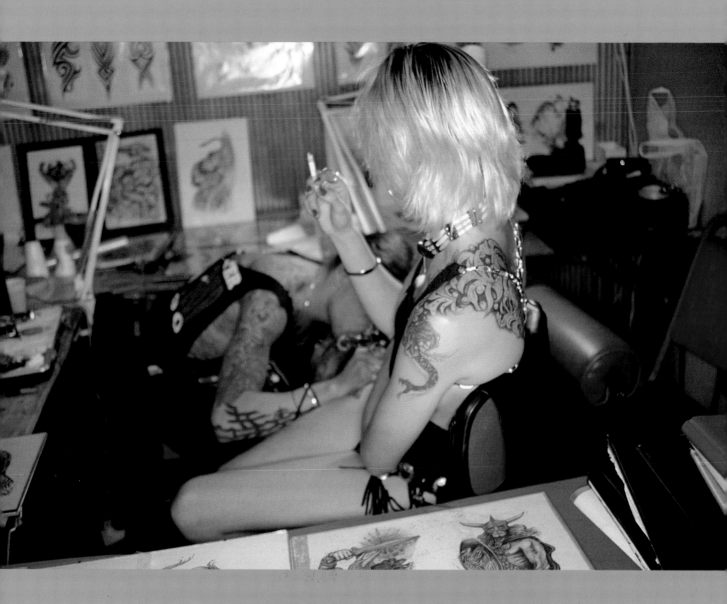

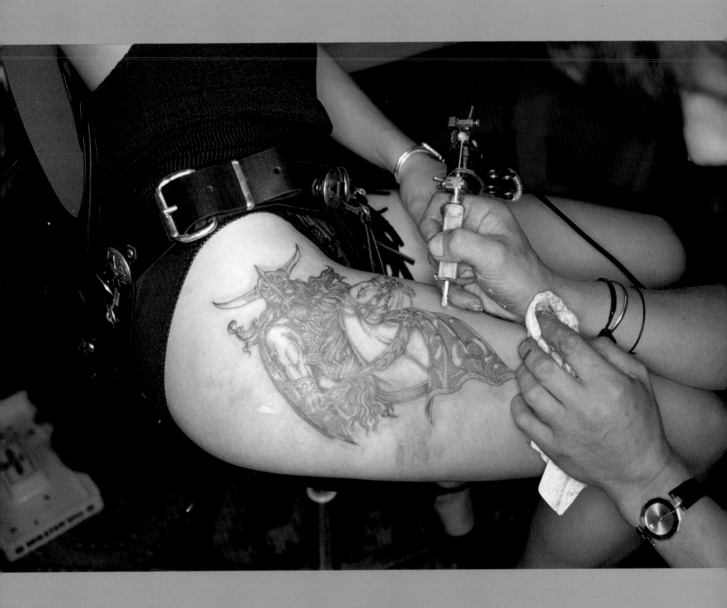

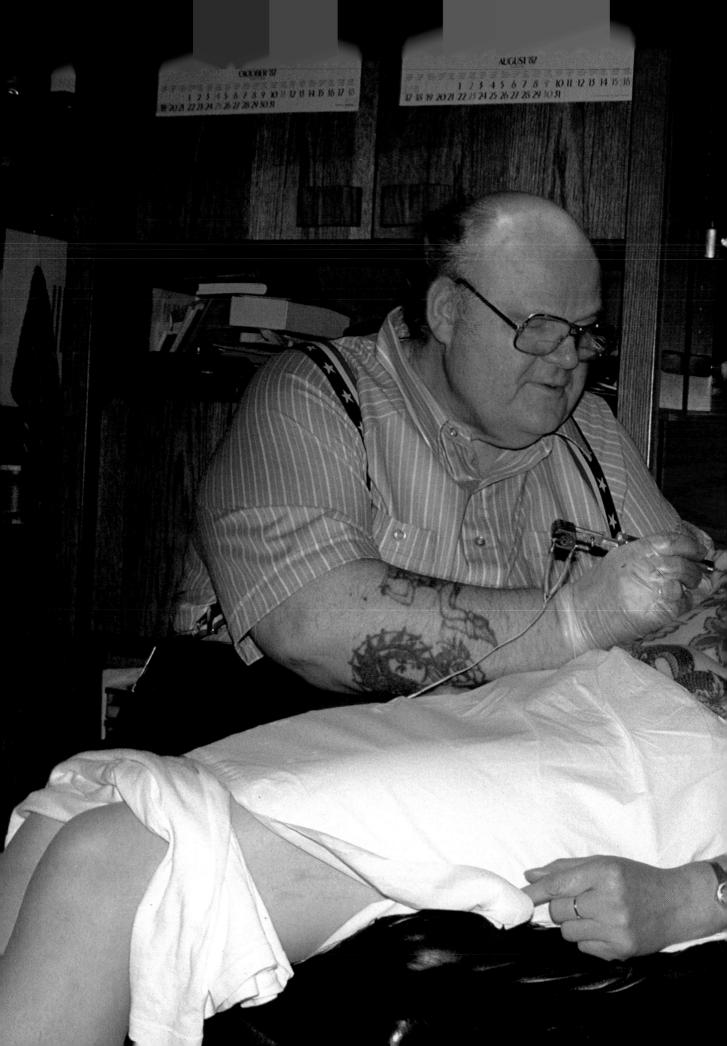

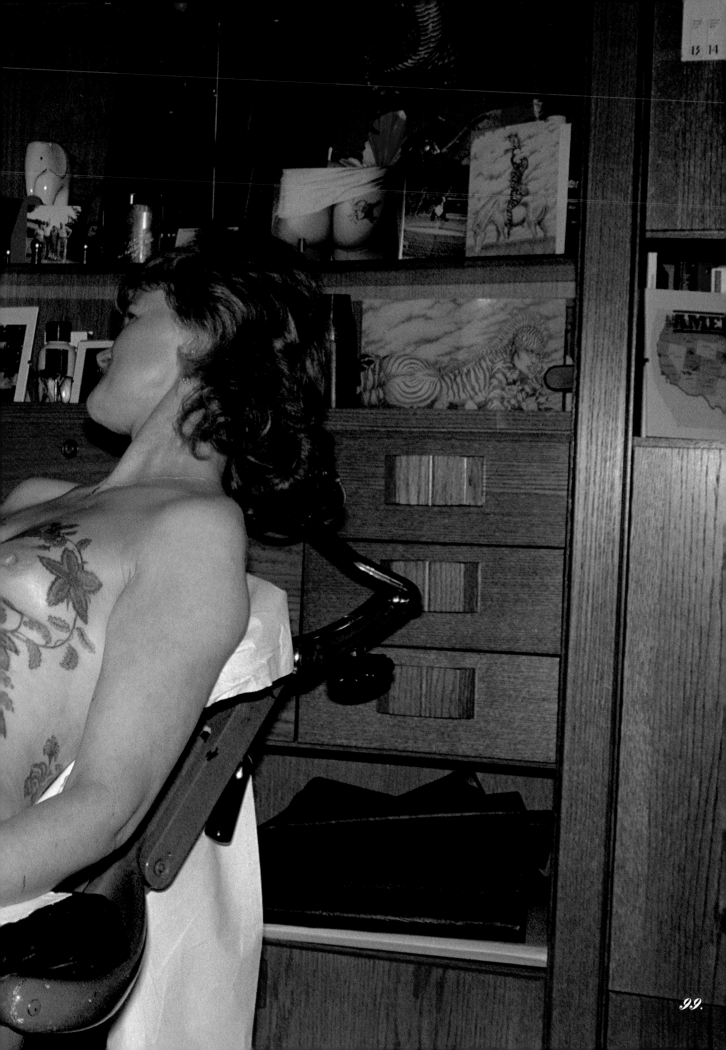

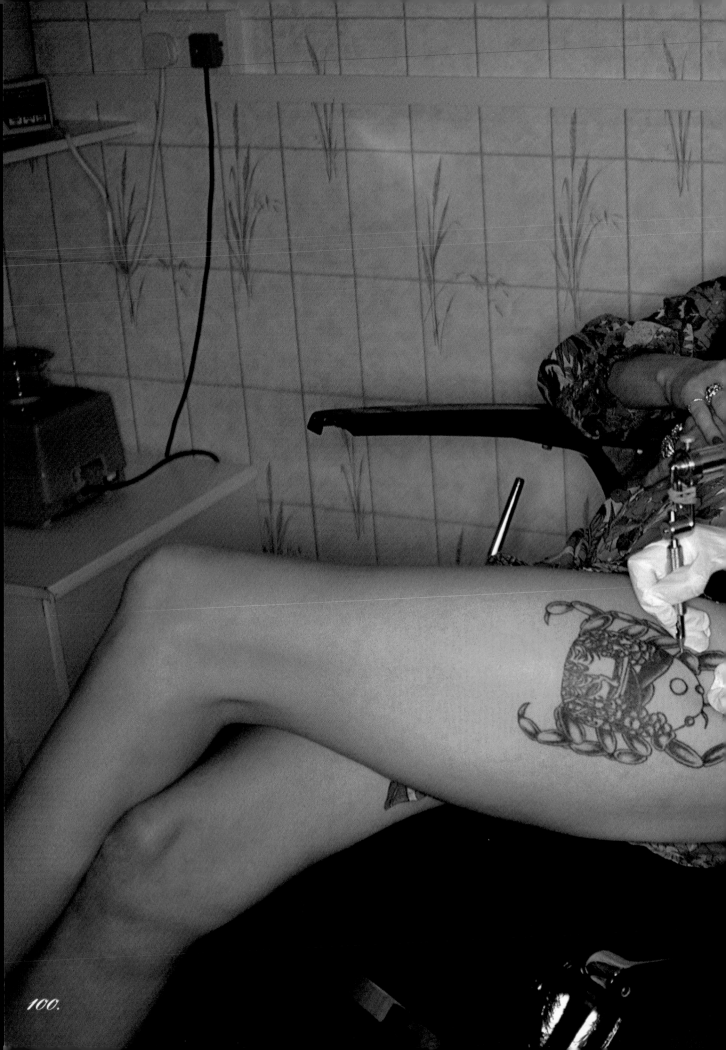

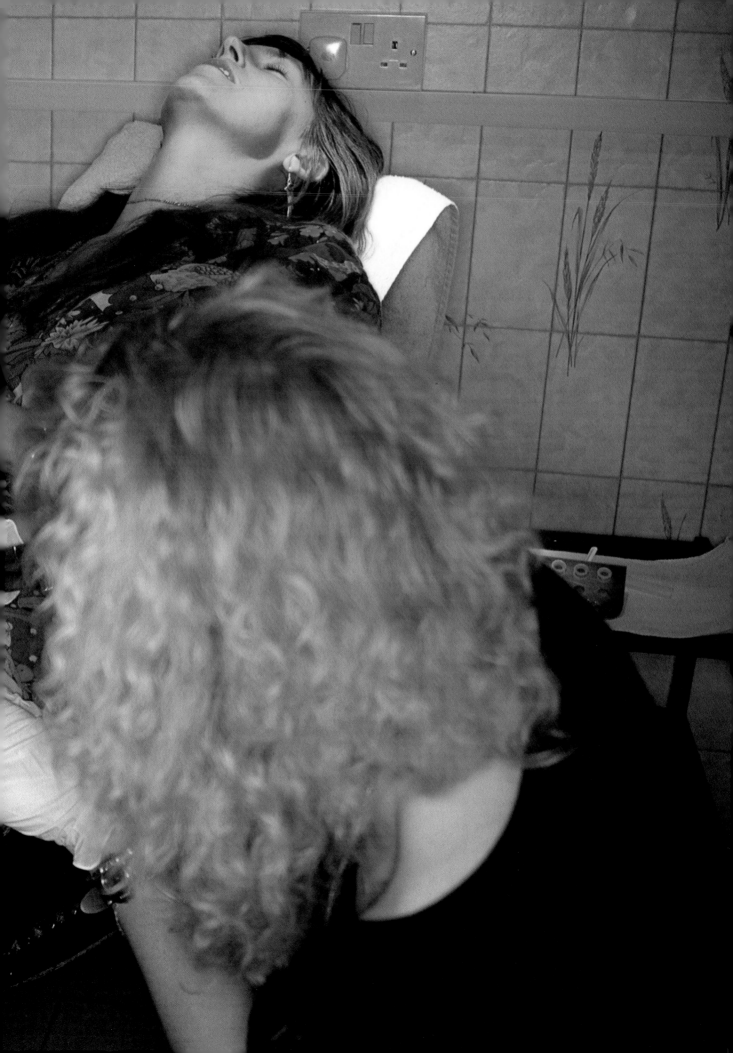

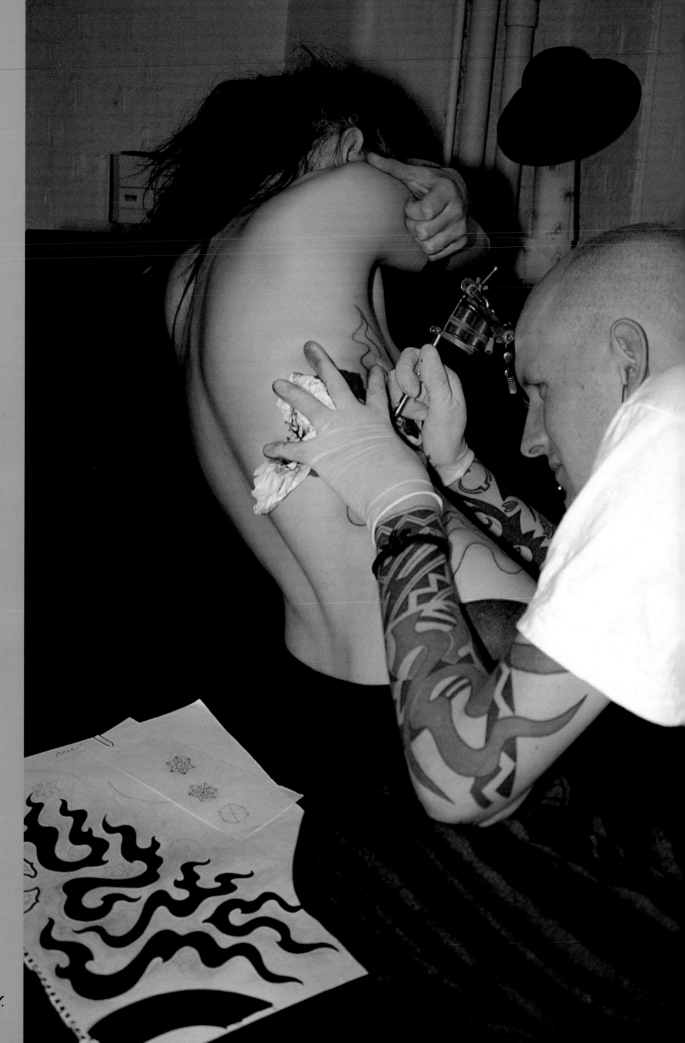

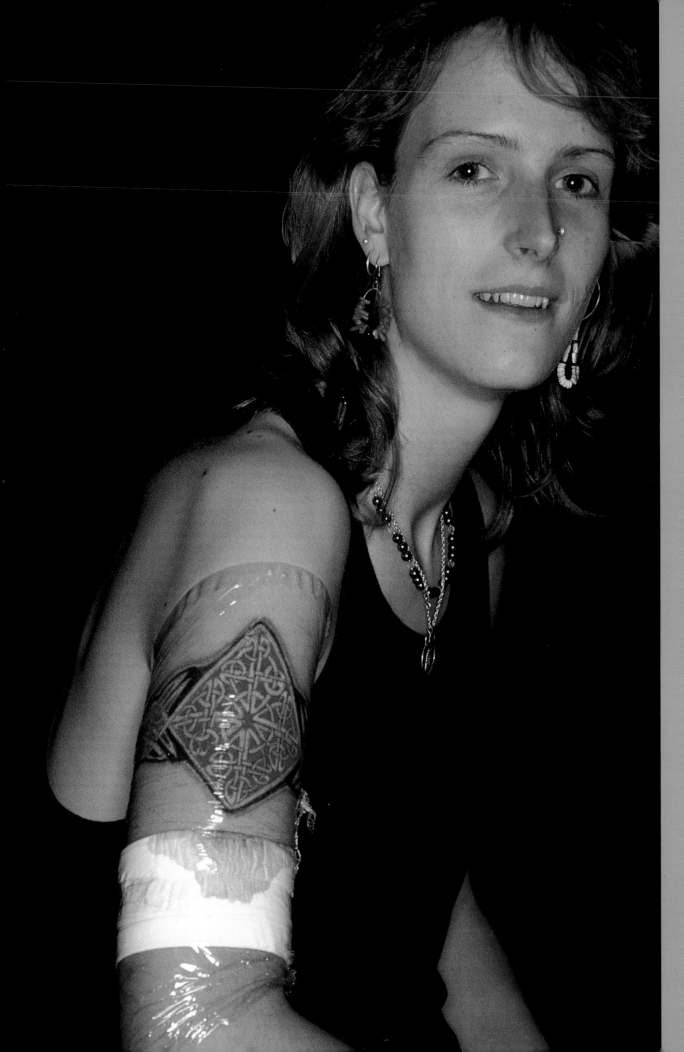

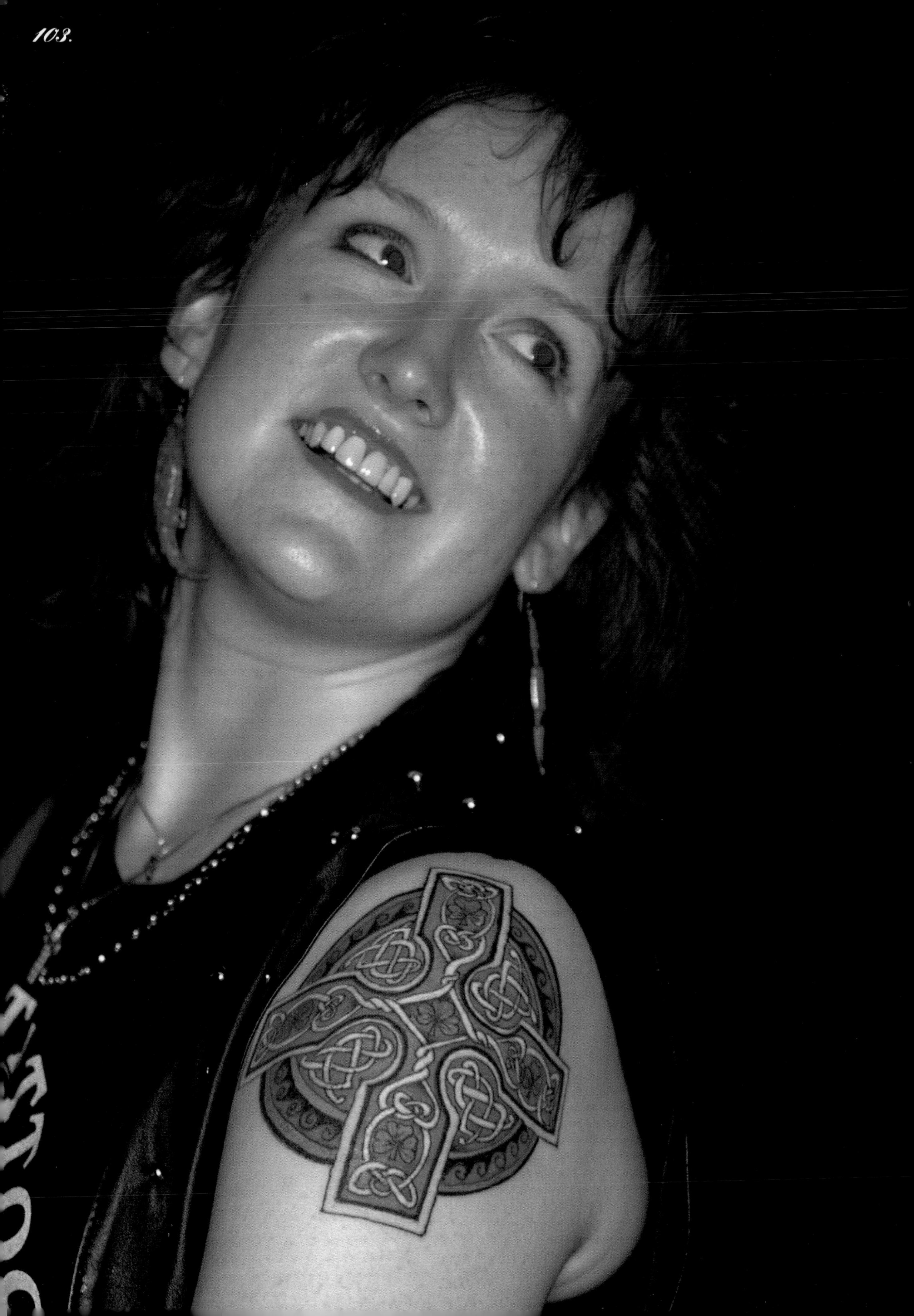

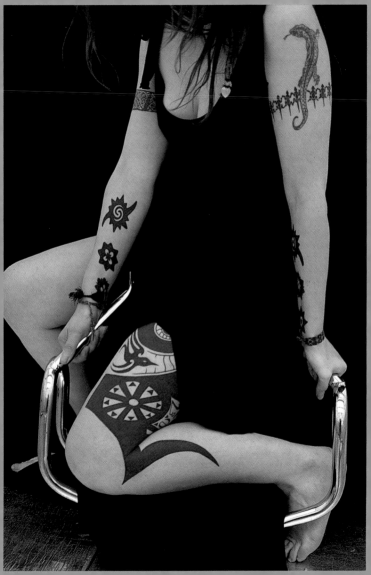

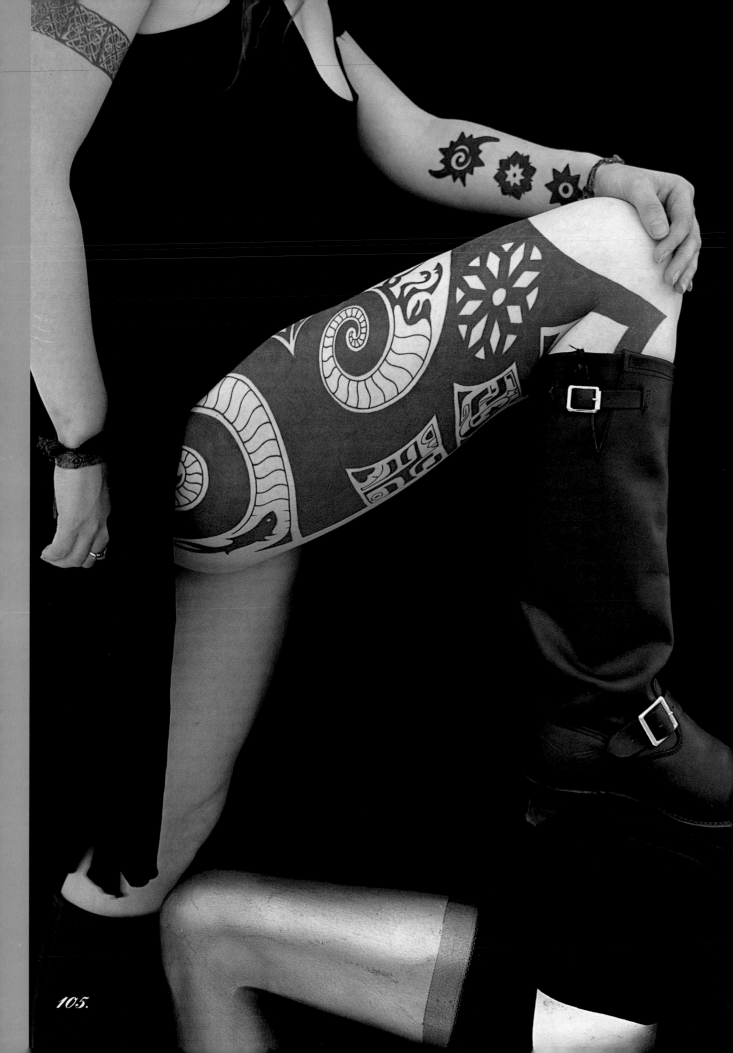

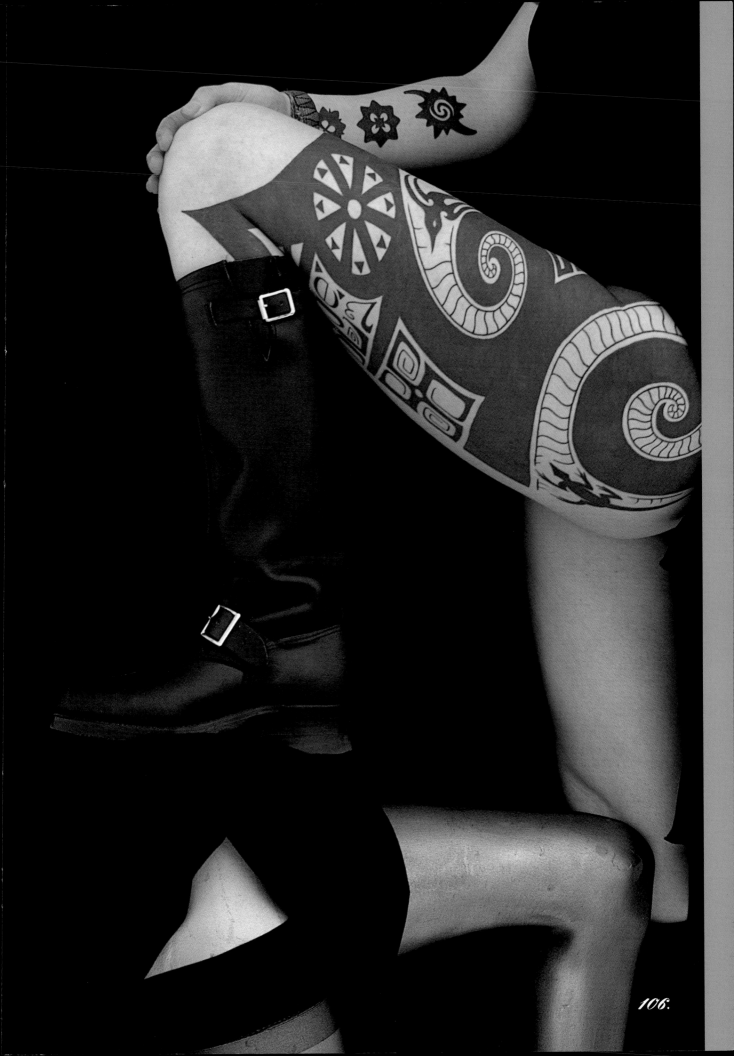

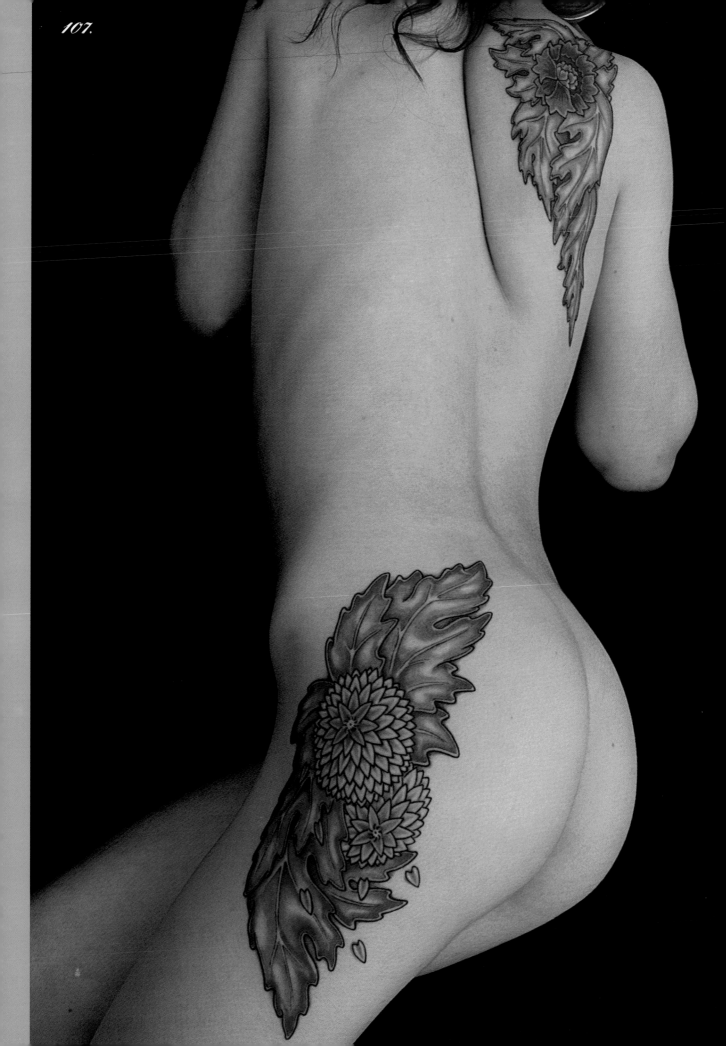

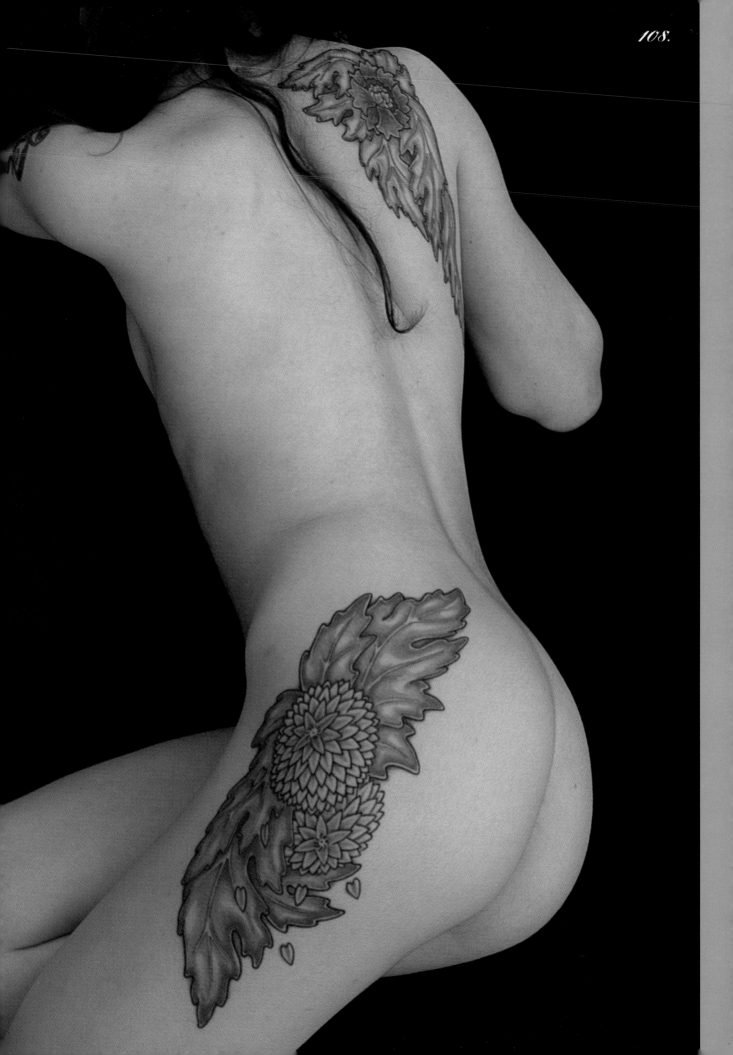

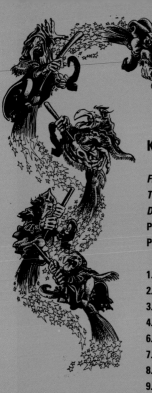

KEY TO PHOTOGRAPHS

Front Cover: Lisa, tattooed by Alex Binnie, London.
Title page: Illustration by Steff Murschetz, Germany.
Dedication page:
Polaroid of Pierrette and Chris by Claudio, Paris, 1991
Polaroid of Lorette Leu - Iban throat tattoo by Felix.

1. Sonja tattooed by Johnny Niesen, Holland.
2. Eileen tattooed by Louis Malloy, Manchester, UK.
3. Anda Maj-Maj, tattooed by John, Copenhagen.
4. & 5. Sabina, tattoos by Erich, Germany.
6. Angela, tattoo by Louis Malloy, UK.
7. Tattoo and photo by Yoshihito Nakano, Yokohama, Japan.
8. Yuki, tattooed by Ian of Reading
9. German Circus advertising posters circa 1920s
10. Cherie, being tattooed by Tin Tin at Dunstable Tattoo Expo, 1991.
11. Inside the tattoo forum at Dunstable.
12. Paul O'Connor at work, Dunstable Expo.
13. Greta being tattooed by Jacky at Dunstable Expo.
14. & 15. Tattoo humour from the Lone Wolf Tattoo Studio, formerly in Luton.
16. Photomontage showing Ainu tattooed woman.
17. Detail from the late Bob Maddison's studio, UK.
18. Detail from George Bone's studio, London.
19. Detail from the late Cash Cooper's studio, London.
20 & 21. Peggi Hurley. Tattoos by Don Nolan - body ; Gill Montie - arms ; Bud Piersen - left foot ; Bill Hannong - right foot ; Marco Pisa - Amsterdam souvenir ; Ken Cameron New Orleans, Winona Martin, Honolulu - eyeliner.
22. & 23. Annabelle Hallas-Moeller, tattoos by Erik Reime, Copenhagen.
24. Lisa and Lisa in action at Chris Wroblewski's tattoo museum, London.
25. Mariz showing tattoos by El Zin, Oberhausen, Germany.
26, 27, 28 & 29. Teena receiving tattoo from Alex Binnie, London.
30. Leopard tattoo by Lal Hardy, London.
31. Iain at the Amsterdam tattoo convention.
32. Betty Altimore, tattoo by Marco Pisa, Bologna, Italy.
33. Val, tattoo by the Dutchman at Skin Deep Tattoo, Maui, USA.
34. Chris, tattoos by Fred Young, UK.

35. Samantha, tattoo by the Dutchman at the Skin Deep Tattoo, Maui, USA.
36. Coco Genziana, tattoo by Berni Luther, Vienna.
37. & 38. Nikki, tattoos by Brent and Amanda, Dunstable.
39. George Burchett's wife.
40, 41 & 42. Clairey the Venusian woman.
43. Kali, tattoos by Vince, Dunstable.
44. Val at the Amsterdam Tattoo Convention.
45. Anda Maj-Maj, tattoos by John Copenhagen.
46. Helle, tattoos by Danny, Copenhagen.
47. Duluneid Bonome, tattoo by Freddy, Sao Paulo, Brazil.
48. Greta McLoud, tattoo by Stuart Wrigley, Glasgow.
49. At the Dunstable Expo, 1991.
50. Ali, Celtic fairy story tattoo by Alan Dean, Luton, UK.
51. Jane Nemhauser, tattoo by Ed Hardy, USA.
52 & 53. Tina, tattoos by Saz Saunders, UK.
54. Misse tattoos by Svend, Copenhagen.
55. Christine, tattoos by Alain, Marseille, France.
56 & 57. Danny in action at the Copenhagen tattoo show 1991.
58 & 59. Tattoos by Erik Reime, Copenhagen. Background illustrations showing Samoan tattoo designs for women by Carl Marquardt, 1899.
60 & 61. American tattoo photographs from the Tattoo History Museum, Oxford.
62. Painless tattooing by Chuck and Dianne, Dagenham, UK.
63, 64, 65 & 66. Lisa tattooing Terry, London, at Lisa Art in the Skin.
67, 68 & 69 At the Dunstable Tattoo Expo, 1991.
70. Lisa, tattoo by Lisa.
71. Tattoo by Kari Barba, Anaheim, USA.
72, 73, 74, 75, 76 & 77. From archives of the Tattoo History Museum, Oxford.
78. Debbie tattooed by Lal Hardy, London.
79 & 80. Kaisu, tattoo by Bugs, London.
81. Tattoo by Spider Webb, photo by Jean Marie Guyaux.
82. Lene tattoos by Erik Reime, Copenhagen.
83 & 84. Vicky, tattoos by Brent, Dunstable, UK.
85. Sam Clay, tattoo by Bob of Ipswich, UK.
86. Leanne Chambers, tattoos by Hanky Panky, Amsterdam.
87. Nancy and child at Skin Deep Tattoo, Honolulu, tattoos by Jack Rudy.
88. Nikki and Lal Hardy, London.

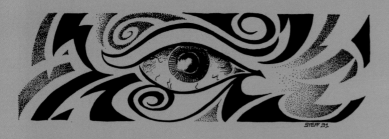

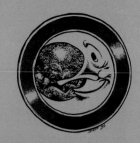

89. Karen, tattoos by Micky Sharpz.
90. Jacki by Micky Sharpz.
91. Denise Evans, willow fairies by Kevin Shercliffe, Staffordshire, UK.
92. Tattoo by Marco Leoni, Brazil.
93. Montage showing Laura from Massachusetts, USA, Japanese girl with tattoo by Lal Hardy, and tattoo business cards.
94. Montage showing tattoo business cards, Japanese tattoos and Flash by Lisa.
95. Chuck being tattooed by Berni Luther at Dunstable tattoo Expo, 1991.
96. Chuck at her studio with completed tattoo by Berni.
97 & 98. Vince at work at the Dunstable Tattoo Expo 1991.
99. Sammy growing flowers at his studio in Frankfurt, Germany.
100. Sue, by Chuck at her Dagenham Tattoo Studio.
101. Alex working on Anne at his London studio.
102. Andi Coppin with fresh tattoo by Pete Larkin, Huddersfield, UK.
103. Mary Larkin, tattoo by Pete Larkin.
104, 105 & 106. Tattoos by Alex Binnie, London.
107. & 108. Lisa, tattoos by Alex Binnie, London.
109. Tattoo design by the late Greg Irons, 1981.
Key illustrations: by Steff Murschetz.
Back cover: Anne, tattoos by Alex Binnie.

STEVE BEARD is a roving intellectual reporter who at the flick of a pen is able to turn his professional attention from subjects as sublime as PM Dawn to the ridiculous like Jean Baudrillard. He contributes regularly to i-D and the **MODERN REVIEW**, and has even appeared as a TV culture pundit, broadcasting live to an audience of millions one twilight evening in Buenos Aires. Over qualified for any regular employment, he remains much too picky about accepting commissions. So far he has resisted the urge to get himself tattooed.

BIBLIOGRAPHY

George Burchett with Peter Leighton. Memoirs of a Tattooist, London, 1958.
Michel de Certeau, The Practice of Everyday Life, London, 1984.
Hanns Ebensten, Pierced Hearts and True Love: A History of Tattooing, London, 1953.
Michel Foucault, Disipline and Punish: The Birth of the Prison, Harmondsworth 1977.
Plinio Martelli, The Tattoo as Art, Padova, 1980.
Arnold Rubin (ed), Marks of Civilization: Artistic Transformations of the Human Body, Los Angeles, 1988.
Clinton Sanders, Customizing the Body: the Art and Culture of Tattooing, Philadelphia, 1989.
Marcia Tucker, Tattoo: the State of the Art, Artform 19, 1981.

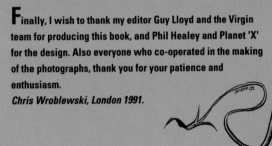

Finally, I wish to thank my editor Guy Lloyd and the Virgin team for producing this book, and Phil Healey and Planet 'X' for the design. Also everyone who co-operated in the making of the photographs, thank you for your patience and enthusiasm.
Chris Wroblewski, London 1991.

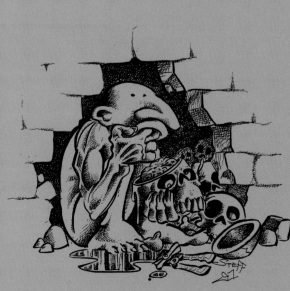

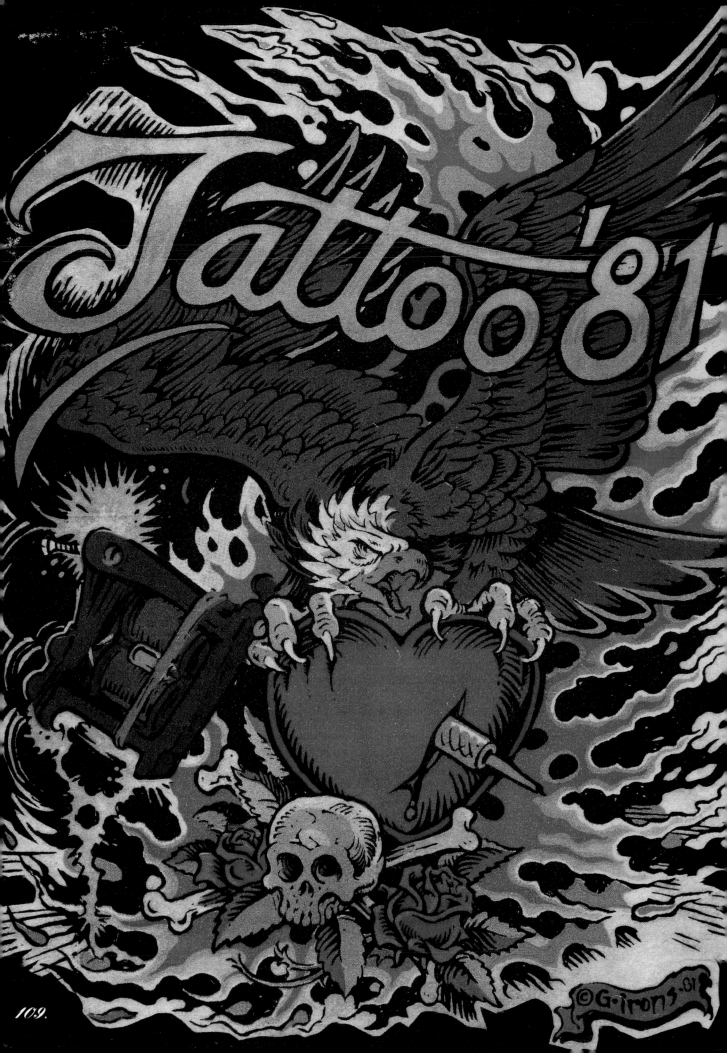